EDIBLE TO INCREDIBLE

AND ALL THINGS BETWEEN:
A NUTRITION TOOLKIT FOR EVERY HOME

SHEEBA MAJMUDAR

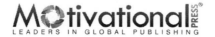

MOtivational PRESS®
LEADERS IN GLOBAL PUBLISHING

Published by Motivational Press, Inc.
1777 Aurora Road
Melbourne, Florida, 32935

www.MotivationalPress.com

Manufactured in the United States of America.

ISBN: 978-1-62865-273-4

CONTENTS

INTRODUCTION

This book has been written for all those people, like me, who find they are placed in a corner with no choices when a loved one is sick. I have met clients and friends alike, who repeatedly give antibiotics or steroids or inhalers to little children, can see the side effects, but feel they have no other choice in the matter. We always have a choice, and this book is to empower individuals to recognize that we all have *many* choices.

There are many diet books, nutrition books on what vitamins and nutrients foods contain, and fitness and health books related to managing or curing a certain condition; this book is *not* about any of that.

I have yet to come across a book for laypeople, where a map or floor plan is laid out as to how to incorporate all aspects of nutritional counseling into their lives.

Many go to Ayurvedic centers or health resorts to sort themselves out for a few days or even weeks, but eventually they come back to living in their everyday urban or suburban environment, with all the pressures and toxicities, and may go back to square one from a health perspective.

This book is a tool for people from all walks of life—those who want to begin to explore, to those who have been following ideas like these for a while and want to discover new options or work on another aspect of their health—there are layers upon layers of information that we can use to work on ourselves. I am trying to offer this book in layers, so that there is something for everyone, even advanced seekers.

Another reason for writing this book was ignited by my own searching and learning and wanting to find a way to help my family—especially my kids, who were prescribed antibiotics by doctors at the drop of a hat. At that point, when your children are not well, and the doctor simply gives you a prescription, you feel helpless and reach for that solution—even if it is not the best in the long haul. All of these things led to my search for answers and inspired me to study nutrition and holistic wellbeing.

I believe that we need to determine the root cause(s) of our issues, and then work on those. Once you treat the roots, the branches and leaves automatically start responding. If you only work on the branches and leaves (your disease and symptoms), getting results may be challenging.

Doctors and medication are required from time to time to address serious situations or acute cases. For most other issues however, there are simple, logical, scientific, and nutritional options that can completely address the health concern at hand.

That is what this book is about. To empower individuals, especially caregivers, who are concerned for their loved ones. The advice is practical for urban living and environments in which stress, travel, toxicity, and food irregularities are ever-present.

People sometimes ask if Ayurveda and Traditional Chinese Medicine would help them.

While they most certainly would, consistency is key. If you are travelling and are unable to boil your herbs or follow the specific diet, then the program will not work. The homeopathic system works for some, but maybe not for all. So is there a middle path that would work for everyone?

There are a few different things I have put together that have worked well for my family and hundreds of clients, as well. As a naturopath and a nutritionist, working tirelessly to help those around me attain wellness, I hope you are able to utilize this book to the fullest extent and experience the results of turning around your health, whether it be from a common cold or cancer.

I write this book in all humbleness that it may assist other people on their own journey of evolution.

FOREWORD

If you have come across this book or this author then chances are you are seeking health answers that haven't been solved by the medical field. You are a seeker of truth and personal discovery. *Edible to Incredible: And All Things Between- A Nutrition Toolkit for Every Home* is your answer. This compilation of valuable and life-changing information is timely and powerful. There are some many products and medications out there that are getting tossed around and tossed out. The information journey you have begun by seeking answers will be rewarded in the pages that follow.

We have been conditioned to believe that all ailments require a diagnosis and eventually a pill for it. Most prescriptions just "cover-up" the symptom and never address the underlying root cause. Much like a loud fire alarm that you place duct tape over to make the noise "go away." When, in fact, we all know if a fire alarm goes off there is usually smoke, that came from a fire, that had something like a little arsonist that started that fire in the first place. Sheeba addresses the root causes of imbalances and illnesses in the body and provides thorough and effective solutions to create a healthy environment.

Sheeba and I have shared the building of a personal journey of transformation and study in Singapore. As a gifted healer and practitioner, she worked to help build a wellness facility clientele with dedication to finding the true imbalance in each individual. By seeing the potential in everyone's healing journey, Sheeba has directed them to tools that are practical and quiet easy. Many of us have been led to believe that healing isn't possible and just to maintain can be tedious, even dangerous measures that we are programmed to believe are necessary. Anyone who takes an interest in the true resolution of their health issues will find powerful inspiration in these pages, in addition to, well researched practical tips that yield marked improvements in lifestyle and well-being.

This book represents the real transformation you can make in your own health and your family. Everyone is different with different issues and Sheeba addresses the root causes so each person can have a customized healing approach. By addressing all points of resistance to change, including emotional and spiritual, Sheeba presents a "whole" plan. She understands resistance, what it's like to lack motivation, to prefer certain tastes, to find clues in your skin, to be skeptical or leery of suggestions that are unappealing or ineffective. This book provides a much-needed wake up call for those that are seeking answers "out of the box."

Sheeba Madjumar's approach challenges many techniques that the health field relies on when they run out of answers. I strongly recommend her approach to all medical professionals, nutritionists and other practitioners looking to be enlightened and increase their insights into health. Sheeba raises the bar in the field by addressing outdated thinking and applications of nutrition.

Kimberly D. Balas, PhD, ND
Author and developer of Nutritional Approach to Blood Chemistry
Product, Research Developer and Practitioner, Casper, WY

HOW BEST TO UTILIZE THIS BOOK

The book you hold in your hand is the first of its kind. It is layered with information that is both user-friendly and doable; it also carries deeper information relevant to healthcare practitioners who already have a good working knowledge in this area.

There are many ways to use this book, but since it is packed with information, it does not need to be read cover to cover in one sitting; it can be read based on what chapter draws your attention first. If someone just wants to start getting healthier, he/she can start with the recommended supplements, tweak his/her diet based on whatever suggestions work best on a personal level, and at some point may want to experiment with embarking on a relevant cleanse. The most important thing to learn from the book is the WHY behind your health challenges.

Once you have understood that, you will find that you have the key to unlock how this book would work for you and how it will unfold. Treat each chapter as an experiment for yourself, just as I have lived this book in its entirety. It is not just knowledge but direct experience being shared, which marks the difference between a reference book and a tool kit. The book is written in layers, as it attempts to bridge the gap between those with a serious interest in the subject, such as healthcare practitioners, and those who may find it as a useful reference point with respect to some specific chapters. The point is not to get bogged down.

Dedicated to my late father, Raj Bhandia who is now my guide.

CHAPTER 1

FOUNDATION

We have all learned biology and the human anatomy and functions in school. So when we get a cough and nose block, we generally know that we have to work on clearing up the lymphatic system. However, we may not remember all the biological reasons for that.

To get you up to speed, we will do a quick review to brush up on what we learned (or should have learned) in school.

THE DETOXIFICATION SYSTEMS AND THEIR CORRESPONDING SUPPORT

Liver: The liver is one of the largest detoxification organs, apart from the skin. It is constantly trying to clean up our system, but it needs specific nutrients and raw materials in order to do so. It handles over five hundred different functions in the body like energy production, metabolism, breaking down hormones, processing drugs, etc. The detoxification happens in two phases. First, it breaks down toxins into harmless components, and next it packages them to be cleared by the lymphatic system. Any lack (of nutrients) or excess (toxins) will prevent complete detoxification, creating a traffic jam or congestion, creating many health issues. The liver also manages blood sugar reactions in the body, and produces the master antioxidant, glutathione, without which we age and fall sick rapidly.

Poor Functioning of Liver: A poor-functioning liver could give rise to many different symptoms, including various skin conditions from acne to psoriasis, migraines and headaches, bloating and flatulence, indigestion, feelings of low energy, poor immunity, depression, and many more.

Support: Complete food-based nutrients with complete vitamins, plant-based minerals, amino acids, and specific antioxidants all work on supporting and clearing the liver. For example, Beyond Tangy Tangerine from Youngevity brand; this is a powder multivitamin mineral supplement derived from 115 fruits and vegetables, that is a powerhouse of highly absorbable nutrients.

Gallbladder: This produces bile and helps to break down or emulsify fats. There is also a correlation to iron highs and lows in a patient. Your gallbladder helps with peristalsis and bowel movements, and a healthy gallbladder is a key to gaining or losing weight.

Poor-Functioning Gallbladder: This would manifest as bloating, poor nutrient absorption leading to anemia, weight gain or loss, chronic constipation, fatigue, high or very low cholesterol, and eventually gallbladder issues result in pain related to gallstones.

Support: A gallbladder cleanse, ox bile salts, and lecithin are all directly going to support this. If you have had your gallbladder removed, this is all the more reason to take ox bile salts with each meal.

Kidneys: This entire system manages the body's electrolytes and water balance while simultaneously removing toxins. The kidneys are usually the most sensitive organs. Chronic dehydration can create a huge stress on this system, which is surprisingly common in today's world.

Poor-Functioning Kidneys: Normally it takes a while to manifest, but the initial signs of poorly functioning kidneys are dark eye circles, water retention, and increased creatinine levels.

Support: Energized water or Kangen water, Himalayan/Celtic sea salt, Gtox Express (a Metagenics supplement that is a super-green powder infused with potent lymph-cleansing herbs), juicing with coriander leaves; parsley leaves; spirulina; and aloe vera all have a cleansing effect on the kidneys.

Skin: The skin is a reflection of the other detoxification systems. It has the largest surface area, therefore the largest detoxification system. All skin issues are related to poor detoxification of all the systems.

Support: Skin is supported by the liver, lymphatic, and kidney detox supports; digestive stomach acid support (take apple cider vinegar with meals); omega3 fats; and manual or electronic tool based lymphatic drainage (see more in later chapters on looking good and feeling good).

Lymphatic System: This system is all over the body, with specific centers that have lymph nodes. The lymphatic system clears the toxins that are thrown out by the liver, and is the main "garbage disposal system" of the body. It also transports hormones, fats, and nutrients to the cells. It has no pump or circulation system so the only way it "moves" is with our own movements.

Poor-Functioning Lymph: Weight loss can be sluggish if lymph is stuck, along with circulation. It could reflect as skin issues, darkened armpits, infections in the groin area, water retention, recurring infections, skin allergies, and/or low or slow sweating.

Support: Lymphatic massage is very helpful, through manual massage or using a handheld device (see the chapter Looking Good, Feeling Good); trampoline jumping; using a power plate machine; along with Gtox Express; detox teas with echinacea, burdock, goldenseal, sarsaparilla, cleavers, and similar teas; as well as homeopathies for lymph, such as lymphomyosot, in either liquid or tablet form.

Digestive System: The digestive system includes the liver and gallbladder. What most people don't know is that it represents over 70 percent of the immune system. The digestive tract is like the Great Wall of China; it prevents infections and pathogens from moving in and prevents undigested food from moving out at the wrong time. This is why all traditional systems of medicine say that all diseases stem from the gut.

Another thing to note is that the stomach produces a strong acid that creates a very acidic pH that helps to break down proteins and absorb minerals, iron, B vitamins, etc. If this is compromised, malabsorption typically occurs.

Poor-Functioning Digestive System: Fortunately, a troubled digestive system will reveal itself loud and clear either by stomachaches, cramps, constipation, diarrhea, etc. Then you can do something about it!

Support: You can support your digestive system by using apple cider vinegar during meals, digestive enzymes, betaine HCl, and liver and gallbladder support as required (see the chapter on Gut for complete support and cleanse).

THE ENDOCRINE SYSTEM

Pineal: This is a master gland that controls the major glands.

Pituitary: Master gland (instructs the entire endocrine system)

Hypothalamus: Master gland (instructs the entire endocrine system)

Thyroid: Metabolism, energy, sex hormones, and weight management. Located in the throat area, the thyroid is very sensitive to toxins.

Adrenals: Located above the kidneys. The adrenals manage the stress response in the body, and produce over 50 different hormones, including sex hormones. They are extremely sensitive to internal and external environmental changes. This gland also manages the body's blood sugar response.

Parathyroid: This gland manages the calcium and vitamin D levels in bones.

Pancreas: The pancreas is responsible for enzyme production to digest food and also to produce insulin, which manages the blood sugar response in the body.

Reproductive system: These glands regulate our sex hormones based on instructions from the master glands.

Now that you have a basic understanding of the major systems, we can move on to understanding how the body works and what we can do to support all systems and keep it efficient and disease free.

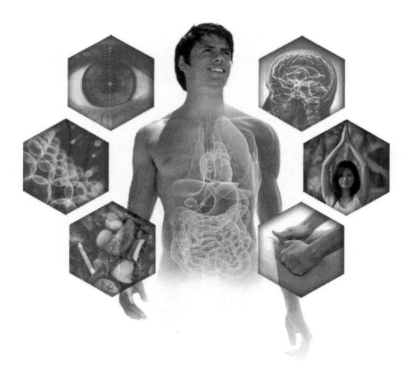

CHAPTER 2

THE BARRIER OF BELIEFS

I t is a documented fact that today we are more exposed to toxins than our ancestors. With planes, mobile phones, computers, pesticides, global transport of food, food storage, GMO foods, and mercury in our food chain, our bodies are overwhelmed with the continuous need to detox. In order to do this, it needs raw materials like vitamins, minerals, amino acids, etc. The higher the toxin exposure, the more nutrients are required. If this equation is tipped, health issues may ensue.

There are many who believe that nature and food should provide everything we need and that supplements are not natural and can cause further harm. They simply do not believe in swallowing more pills in the name of health.

I think it is very important to be cautious about what you put into your body, as we are all architects of our own health.

When building a house, you need to make sure all the raw materials used are of good quality, otherwise the house may have shaky foundations, and we know what happened when the Big Bad Wolf blew the pigs houses down.

Similarly, what we choose to put into our bodies as raw material goes into creating each cell. If we choose to put in junk, our cells are created with junk. Don't expect the body that is fed junk to support you in times of stress.

Families Today: Pets, kids, men, and women all form the family. Many men have constant stress at work, balancing accounts, and in the roles of husband, father, and son. Women now have resorted to multitasking with work, home, kids, acting as entrepreneur, wife, daughter, and mother. Adults' stress affects their children too, as well as school stress, and social peer pressures to boot. Pets are exposed to the health beliefs of the family. For example, if the family is vegetarian, they will normally feed vegetarian food to their dogs. This may not be the right diet for the dog, and it limits the pets' diet.

Barrier of Beliefs: Similarly, our belief systems play a major role in our food choices, our health care choices, and how we perceive illness and health. If you believe that your parents had cancer so it is inevitable that you will get it because of genetics, the possibility becomes very real. If you realize that we all have cancer genes, but it is *up to you* to switch it on or off, then you are truly taking responsibility for your health. This is also the role of epigenetics, where now genes are not seen as the end all, but instead research has shown that our genes respond to our environment, both physical and mental. This is why a healthy diet, exercise, and meditation all do wonders for most people.

Once you take responsibility for the health issues that come up, do not believe in dead ends. That is where true health and healing starts. Know that if it has come, then it can also go. Your body is just trying to get your attention for something it lacks. Many people may have colon cancer, and can have a general treatment protocol, but their unique biochemistry means that each one will have specific gaps to fill in, so protocols will eventually need to be customized. There is no one-size-fits-all solution.

I have worked with many clients who are personal trainers with great bodies, flexible clients who are yoga teachers, who eat vegan, raw foods, or are vegetarians. These people may look good in a variety of poses, but they are not necessarily the healthiest of clients. In fact, I was always shocked to find that their assessments were not reflective of their lifestyle at all. This made me wonder what really makes or breaks a person's health. The belief system is one of them, and so are exercise and diet; these two factors have the ultimate power of turning around health. There is definitely a third element, which I will mention later on. Not wanting to harm animals, take supplements, or trust in a doctor's prescription are all beliefs that can limit the healing process. The best bet is to be nonjudgmental, and most importantly, open-minded.

I would like to share a heart-warming story of my client here. She came to me after countless rounds of fertility drugs for over two years. She had gone to see an IVF specialist who, horrified at her track record, point blank stated that it would be difficult to have a successful IVF as she had PCOS (Polycystic Ovarian Syndrome), and a poor track record with the fertility drugs. His advice for her was to lose weight in order to gain a better chance for a successful IVF. She had tried many times to lose weight without success. Then, she decided to seek professional help.

That's where I came in the picture. She not only lost nine kilos in two months, but she continued to eat right and lose three more kilos totaling up to a healthy twelve kilos down. The following month she was *naturally pregnant*! No drugs, no IVF–she carried the baby full term and now has a healthy child. What really changed? As her body began to lose weight and become healthy again, her hope and belief in herself, her body, and the capacity to heal changed. The doctors had all told her she would have PCOS for life and that chances for IVF success were slim. In her medical check-up she was declared PCOS-free. Her negative burden/belief lightened as she did—and a little miracle was born.

There are recorded "miracles" that take place during hypnotherapy. Have you heard of one of those? Where the person is hypnotized to believe the burns on his or her hand will heal at the count of three—and the skin actually heals. There are many such real cases. How does it happen? Our body is made of liquid crystals that store information as light (energy). Now, according to quantum physics, matter is actually nothing but space. The only reason we see an object is because our consciousness has created that reality; the "space" is held together by atoms created by thoughts, and yes, beliefs.

I know this is a lot to digest, and would pointedly mean that we create our reality here on earth. Yes. Read more about this in *Biology of Beliefs* by Dr. Bruce Lipton and *The Secret of the Flower of Life* by Drunvalo Melchizedek. Also read some of Gregg Braden's amazing eye-opening books, such as *Spontaneous Healing of Belief*, which reveals the power of the human mind and our evolution on this planet. These books will open your eyes and change your beliefs.

So, the only thing that limits you from true healing is your beliefs.

You will be exploring more in this book that will require you to keep an open mind.

I am a 44 yr old woman from Jakarta, Indonesia. I was diagnosed with Hashimoto disease (autoimmune) by my gynecologist in 2014. I was determined to look for an alternative treatment for this and stumbled upon Sheeba's website in 2015 April. I flew in to Singapore to consult her. She checked my blood tests and customized a plan for me that was doable for me. in Sep

2015, I did another blood test with an endocrinologist who surprised me by saying I no longer had Hashimoto's! My doctor had mentioned that there was no medicine to reduce high antibodies (which was my case earlier) and it normally is for life. But i am living proof that this statement is not 100% correct as i am certain that upon following Sheeba's recommendations that really healed me, and for which I am grateful. Thank you Sheeba.

Phin Phin S, 44 Yrs, Female.

CHAPTER 3

FOOD FOR THOUGHT

Dogs are fed packaged foods that resemble real food. There are more questionable things in dog food now that would shock any pet lover. There are many articles on dog foods tested for this with evidence.

Then you have kids and teenagers eating fast food that doesn't even rot—this can be seen in a YouTube video of a burger from McDonald's that remains the same for three days. High in trans fats, sugar, corn syrup, artificial sweeteners, dyes, preservatives, hidden chemicals, and heavy metals, our food is no longer edible. What about water? First-world and third-world countries alike have water filled with hormone disruptors, heavy metals, toxins, fluoride, and some is even treated sewage water… you get the picture.

The soil in which our plants grow is contaminated with toxic illegal pesticides, like DDT. The air pollution is at alarming levels, especially if you are living in China or India, where the amount of pollution is so great it is equivalent to smoking a few cigarettes a day!

Even if you live in a fairly clean country, the effects of radiation from

Fukushima and other disasters affect the food chain, oceans, fish, and soil, and this is seen for centuries down the food chain, as we saw in the Chernobyl disaster.

There may be a solution to all these issues, but it's not happening too soon. We can't stop eating and breathing and start planting our own foods (although it is a good idea!), so what is the solution if there is no end to the problem?

First, let's look at what foods are good for us.

Real Foods: My definition of real food is anything made by a human versus a corporation. Therefore, packaged food is not defined as real food. As harsh as this may sound, even healthy foods may not be "real": can you compare your mum's chicken soup to the store-bought one? No contest.

Every time you choose real foods, you choose better nutrition, period. The same goes for your pets.

Carbohydrates: Vegetables, greens, and fruits that are not processed (for example, not in a can), are sound carbohydrate food choices. Lentils, legumes, and whole-grain cereals that are unprocessed (for example, rice made into noodles is more processed than brown rice itself) are healthy. Carbohydrates are important for all meals. The evil "carb" that people are concerned about are the refined foods. Children need to have a higher healthy carbohydrate diet as their metabolism is high and they are in the growth phase. But even kids need to stay away from harmful carbs like sugar and refined foods.

Good Fats: These are the oils that are cold-pressed (unrefined), for example, extra virgin olive oil, coconut oil, grape seed oil, sesame oil, and other nut oils. The key here is *unrefined.* The much-advertised heart-healthy oils like sunflower are in reality the ones that actually cause more damage and increase rates of heart disease. The oils need to be cold-pressed and unrefined to truly benefit. Most of these oils get damaged with heat, so cooking with them is not appropriate. The best way to use them is to create a mixture of extra virgin olive oil, cold-pressed grape seed oil, red palm oil (high in nutrients, especially vitamin A, hence the color), coconut oil, and any other saturated oil like cocoa butter, ghee, or lard.

Most people are shocked at the mention of ghee or coconut oil, as they are often considered the "bad guys" or saturated fats. In reality, these are fats that are not oxidized or damaged in high heat, and therefore are the best oils to mix with olive or grape seed, as they increase the smoking point of the other oils and can safely be used for cooking, stir frying, or even deep frying.

Proteins: It is a scientific fact that our body needs only 0.8 grams of protein per kilogram of body weight. That means significantly less protein consumption than what most people assume!

This is a favorite question asked by many of my clients, as more people are advised to follow a higher protein diet to lose weight and stay healthy. All manner of proteins are generally healthy, except for the extracts or isolated proteins found in protein drinks. The most bioavailable (best absorbed by the body) is actually a vegetarian protein source that's an ancient Aztec grain called quinoa. Quinoa beats chicken and fish as the *numero uno* protein.

Amaranth comes close to quinoa as well, and is a similar grain. Almost all media will inform you to eat more protein, and this is overemphasized by most. Remember that protein is an amino acid—it is acidic in nature. So too much can't be a good thing, as our body pH is actually alkaline. Even toxins are acidic in nature.

But how much is good enough? For most, including athletes, a fistful of protein per meal is enough. According to the nutritional scientists, athletes need only 2.4 grams of protein more than the average person! That is just half a teaspoon of amino acids we are talking about! But remember, you are *not* what you eat, but what you *absorb*. So if your digestion is compromised, then you will not see the results you desire from food alone.

A great example of shattering this protein myth is Ultra Man Rich Roll, who is a vegan, and eats only plant proteins and real foods. He is a lean endurance runner who inspires others. Another person I admire is Skip Archimedes, who is a two-time gold medal winner (UK) in gymnastics. He has an amazing body and, more importantly, is vibrantly healthy. He has a great following and is an inspiring leader for people who want to take charge of their own health by going vegan. He conducts courses on health and healing all over the world.

Anti-Nutrients: As we have become global citizens and many have moved away from their traditional foods, there is a price that we pay. We have convenience foods, fast foods, and refined foods that are frequently a part of our week. We may not be able to get rid of them so easily, but it makes a vast difference if you do. When they are a part of your diet, they are devoid of nutrients, and instead, are termed as *anti-nutrients* as they actually take away nutrients from your body in order to be digested. So each time you eat them, you are depleting the good store of nutrients.

Refined foods tend to behave like sugar in the body: they increase insulin levels rapidly at the same time as they deplete the body of nutrients, not to mention they take longer to digest, which can easily lead to increased fermentation in the gut.

The other anti-nutrients are the hormones in the chicken or milk, the pesticides in greens, and other FDA-approved additives, like food colorings and preservatives. Pure foods are hard to find, but that is why eating organic is not about gaining more nutrients, but instead it's about what you are *not* putting into your body—toxins.

Anti-nutrients are also foods that you are allergic to. Walnuts may be a great health food, but if your body reacts to it, it is identifying it as a toxin. So staying away from foods that cause major or minor food sensitivities can also improve health. This means that anything can be an anti-nutrient—it is body-and person-specific!

Did You Know?

Canola oil is linked to lung cancer. Using refined oils is not an option—so switch to healthy fats like extra virgin coconut oil, red palm oil, ghee, lard, cold-pressed grape seed oil, or nut oils.

Organic Lifestyle: An organic lifestyle is not possible for all, but there are definitely some considerations to make. Our shampoos, creams, lotions, face potions, hand soap, nail polish, and makeup all contain carcinogens or hormone disruptors. The fact is that they may be in small amounts, yes, but a mixture of carcinogens create a powerful synergy which one toxin cannot. It is this multiple-toxin onslaught that one needs to try and avoid. So where you can, choose clean personal-care brands, which you use every single day on your body. The skin's outer layer is dead, but it is an effective transdermal carrier of nutrients, hormones, or toxins. So be wary, cautious, and investigate before you buy. Minimizing toxins is part of keeping and staying healthy.

Trans Fats: Another must-avoid in this war against anti-nutrients is trans fats, which are in the form of hydrogenated vegetable oils, partially hydrogenated vegetable oils, shortening, or simply labeled as trans fats. (Please note that shortening is a manmade fat whereas lard is the fat off any meat, which is the real deal.) They are a manufacturer's dream, as trans fats create a longer shelf life of all baked or fried goods, preventing spoilage and extending expiration dates as well. Just because a label reads 0 grams trans fat doesn't mean it doesn't have any; it just means that the product may contain less than 0.5 grams of trans fat per serving. So, that is still trans fat! We don't want *any* in our food. The reason that it is the worst food choice is simply because it is a manmade synthetic that studies are now recognizing as the main culprit in clogging arteries and increasing all chronic diseases, especially cardiovascular, even in children as young as fifteen years old. In one study, it was discovered that the trans fats were just moving around in the bloodstream; as the body does not recognize it as a food, it does not know what to do with it. It takes one hundred days for that trans fat to be deposited or substituted for fat in our body, creating great health hazards.

The Right Diet: There is a lot of controversy regarding the ongoing research, which attempts to define a diet that is perfect for humans. There are arguments that we are omnivores, so we should eat meat and grains, and others that reveal a vegetarian approach is the healthiest one. Yet another says going vegan or paleo is the best. There are also studies being done on tribes that have people over one hundred years old in the pink of health who eat organic, drink mountain water, and grow and cook their own food.

I always wondered as a nutritionist, what the right answer is. After seeing hundreds of clients from different cross sections, cultures, food habits, and lifestyles, and reviewing many blood test reports, I find there is no right answer. I have clients who are gluten sensitive and for years have not eaten any gluten. One such client did her food allergy test after three years of being gluten free and was a little devastated that her food allergies now showed that she was allergic to rice! What does that mean? Is gluten-free a healthy diet? Not necessarily.

Unless we are working on the root issues, in this case it was working on her leaky gut, no matter what she ate, eventually her digestive system and immune systems would get sensitive to foods eaten repeatedly. This vicious cycle can continue unless she works on healing her gut lining. Please see the digestive chapter for details on how to support a leaky gut.

I also find that if a person has been going heavy on meats, then his/her body will do very well if he/she switches to a heavy plant-based diet for a while. If a person has more grains in his/her diet, like many Asians, then cutting that out for a while may ease the digestive response in that person. So everyone's criteria for switching foods or cleansing would be based on deviating from their everyday foods. Try it!

I also find it appalling that children are still taught a very archaic and outdated food pyramid model in school. I would like to share what I think would be relevant for almost everyone and is an eye opener to most people:

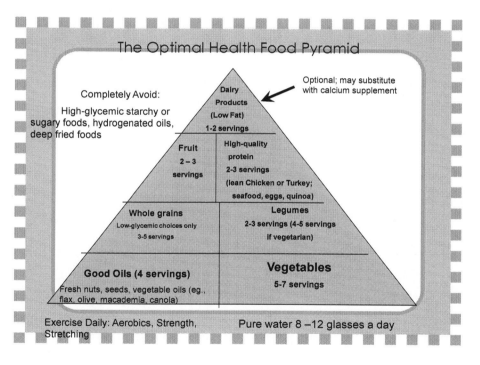

This pyramid comes as a shock to many as it's almost the opposite of the original! Good fats and vegetables are the baseline here? Really? Try following this food pyramid and see what happens! Your health will be transformed forever, and you will not need to do another diet again.

The Secret to What Is Right for You: I have found that what is right for one person may not be right for another. Some common sense here—if a person eats a lot of meat daily, and he switched to eating more vegetables and fruits, would it benefit his health? Yes, the change in diet would do him a world of good. Similarly, if someone consuming sugar daily was asked to quit, would it benefit his health? It most definitely would. If someone having six cups of coffee a day were to reduce or cut intake, they would feel much better after the withdrawal symptoms are gone. Tweaking the diet based on the person's current food consumption can be the clue as to which way he should go with regards to a beneficial diet. He does not have to follow one of the many fad diets in the market.

In general, we are a part of a part of Mother Earth, and the food that is right for us is entirely based on our geography and weather pattern. It is based on harmony with nature, as to what is grown and available on that land, in that season. In the early days, based on geography and season, crops were planted and animals were hunted. This also determined how physically active we were; man would be busy with outdoor activities in the summer that would become minimal during the cold winter.

Now with people on the move, food transport and no dearth of food in all seasons, this is a forgotten and lost condition for food choices. If you are a fisherman, you will eat fish. Can you ask the fisherman to become a vegetarian?

A personal realization has been that as intelligent humans, we are capable of adapting to different geographies (unlike animals) and weather patterns—so we need to get judgment out the door. There are many, including myself, who have judged "meat eaters" as having a poor sense of choice, against spiritual practices. But after years of searching for the truth, I got proof in black and white that as long as we eat while respecting nature, we are in synch with the universe. I found vegans and vegetarians (including yoga teachers!) to generally turn up with poor assessment results, similar to the results of those who abused their bodies!

Hmm… what was going on here? My personal explanation is that the more conditions we place on our body and judgments we have of others, the more we create very rigid patterns that can be demanding of us. We need to be more like a flowing river and go with what comes, or like the zen comparison of a resilient bamboo that can bend and sway with the wind lest it snap.

If you have health ailments and are looking for a solution, there are incomparable studies that show that a plant-based diet that is free from wheat and dairy and plentiful with juices (raw foods) can turn around health in days. Yes, not months, but days. If you can adopt this even as an experiment or detox to see how you feel, it would be a transformation. However, don't forget to continue getting in your daily reliable supplements (I will speak about this in later chapters) as well, along with some outdoor sunshine where you can connect with nature.

As we are a part of nature, we need to learn from it and be a part of it. This is also a challenge living in an urban environment, and henceforth the need for this book.

I am not asking a religious vegetarian to open his mind and start eating meat; my point is that our rigid compartmentalization or calcified judgments can create health challenges for us. I myself was born vegetarian and can't get myself to eat meat. But we do need to be open to taking nourishing supplements to fully support our bodies.

Good Fats: These are essential for all cellular health, hormones, and metabolism. "Good fats" means direct consumption of the fats in the food like nuts, seeds, avocadoes, fatty fish, etc., in contrast to oil that is used for cooking.

Vegetables: All and any—the more colors the vegetables have the better—so choose a rainbow and juice it, soup it, steam it, or have it as a raw salad…any way is good.

Proteins Mixed: Choose from a variety of proteins—remember that meats are heavy and hard-to-digest proteins, and go for leaner white meat from fish and chicken. Quinoa is the best vegetarian source, along with amaranth, legumes, lentils, and brown rice.

Whole Grains: Choose a variety here as well: millets, whole grains like brown rice, steel-cut oats or rolled oats (not quick cooking oats), whole wheat, etc.

Dairy: This is optional, as the calcium in milk is no longer bioavailable due to the pasteurization and homogenization of milk. Cheese and yogurt are better options to attain calcium. Many cultures do not consume milk, but due to westernization, this is rapidly changing.

Sweets, Alcohol: These are optional and are considered empty calories. In fact, they are anti-nutrients that take away nutrients from the body. Consumer beware.

Did you know?

Red palm oil, traditionally used in Africa, is touted as *the* most nutritious oil, even better than coconut oil! It is saturated oil that is reddish in color because of its high vitamin A content, in the form of beta-carotene and lycopene. It has a high content of tocotrienols, or vitamin E, as well, so it is all in all a very high nutrient-packed oil that does not oxidize with high temperature cooking.

I was referred to Sheeba by my cardiologist. Having been diagnosed with hypertension since I was 26, the diagnosis on high cholesterol and hypothyroid also kicked in after childbirth.

I had a sudden weight increase. I started seeing Sheeba and in a matter of 3 months, my blood test results were all normal — cholesterol, thyroid, high uric acid and even my blood pressure. I have already reduced some of my medications thanks to Sheeba's health plan. Now I feel rejuvenated and very much in the pink of health."

Lalithaa M, 35 yrs.

CHAPTER 4

COUNTING NUTRIENTS NOT CALORIES

There are many who still believe in counting calories to maintain weight and even have mobile apps to tell them how much they ate at each meal. This approach completely misses the point of *what* you are putting in your mouth. Remember, you are an architect. If your body is your house, then you want to be using the best-quality materials for the construction of your home.

Calorie counting means you can eat a bar of chocolate for lunch and it won't matter as long as you stick to the day's calorie intake, as it's a number. This will create a healthy relationship with food and healthy options.

Super Foods: In today's deficient world of nutrients, anti-nutrients, and toxic exposure, super foods have to become the household norm.

"Superfoods" are all foods that contain good carbohydrates, proteins, fats, and fiber, as well as some potent antioxidants. Some super examples are listed here:

Coconut (yes, the humble coconut is my number-one choice), raw cacao (chocolate), wolfberries, moringa leaves, chlorella, spirulina, different algae, seaweeds, quinoa, sea vegetables, noni, mangosteen, wheat grass, barley grass, and many more that are still being discovered.

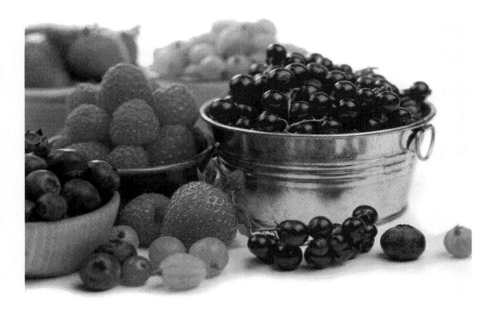

I find that a lot of children today have to wear glasses despite their parents not having any. High use of computers is one reason, but another reason behind that is the constant exposure to radiation. In order to counter radiation effects from electronic devices, we need plenty of antioxidants that can buffer that. This can work not only as a preventive measure, but it can also reduce or reverse your eyeglass number.

We as humans are originally from the sea, as are all organisms. The sea is the primordial soup from which all organisms evolved. All food in the manner of fish, seaweed, and sea vegetables are highly nutritious and dense in minerals. The sea plants are especially high in iodine, an essential mineral for us all, which I will be mentioning in a later chapter. Now you know why the Japanese Okinawans are one of the healthiest and longest living population on the planet!

Super water: Water is the most taken for granted nutrient, and yet, it creates the biggest impact in the body and a sense of wellbeing that no other nutrient can. Over the hundreds of clients I have seen and transformed (with respect to their blood tests), I have found well over 80 percent to be dehydrated at a cellular level. This is not the same thing as orally hydrating three liters a day. The question is again: Are you absorbing it? Sounds quite ridiculous! Not absorbing water?

But there are many who still feel thirsty, have dry skin, and need to keep running to the toilet after drinking water. It just doesn't seem to stay inside long enough. So what's going on here?

Let's start from the beginning. If your toxic load (pesticides, chemicals, heavy metals) has reached a point where it is higher than the body's detoxification capabilities due to lack of raw materials (vitamins, minerals, amino acids) for detoxification, then all cells tend to get full of metabolic waste. The extra-cellular space (space between two cells) is like the road we drive on. Since the cell is full, the water tends to hang around in the extra-cellular space, along with nutrients and hormones, all vying to communicate and get into the cell. There is already a traffic jam inside the cell, and now there is one outside the cell as well. This starts to create cellular dehydration and cell insensitivity, which eventually gives rise to insulin resistance (an instance where the body produces insulin but the cells don't respond to it).

It is worth knowing that all chronic diseases (high blood pressure, diabetes, autoimmune issues, etc.) have one thing in common: cellular dehydration.

The answer to this dehydration would definitely be to clean up the cells, as only drinking more water will not resolve the situation. The simplest way to create a turnaround is to introduce the body to restructured water, or "super water". This water is void of fluoride and organic waste.

There are many types of water filters that claim to produce restructured water, but I have witnessed many medical and immediate clinical benefits with Kangen water, a 40 year old Japanese water filter system.

It is a system worth investing in, but in order to do that we need to understand the basic principles of water.

First, there are many benefits of proper hydration:

1.   Mental well-being
2.   Improved mood
3.   Improved bowel movements
4.   Improved sleep
5.   Improved oxygenation
6.   Improved circulation
7.   Improved detoxification
8.   Increased energy
9.   Increased mental alertness
10.   Increased stamina
11.   Decreased headaches
12.   Decreased muscle cramps
13.   Balanced weight

With these numerous benefits in mind, what we need to know is how the restructured water can achieve cellular hydration while normal water cannot. Almost all of us are more acidic than we should be, although we ideally need to be alkaline. The more acidic we are, the more likely we are to develop diseases. The restructured water is alkalinizing and is naturally high in antioxidants. (You can do your own research later to compare or understand how it works). Normal tap water or bottled water is oxidizing (ages you), and is mostly acidic to neutral pH. The Kangen goes up to a pH of 9.5. Normal water also has water molecules that tend to coalesce in groups of up to 120 molecules clustered together. This acts like one large molecule, which makes it difficult to move in and out of the cell if said cell is already full of metabolic waste.

While the high antioxidants are anti-aging and prevent sickness, the "restructured" water means that these large water clusters have been broken down to just 6 molecules of water as opposed to 120 (effectively lowering surface tension). This makes the water permeable in even small cellular spaces, creating true hydration for the first time. In fact, most people after drinking the restructured water even for a day feel the effects of a detox, ranging from tiredness, to fatigue, increased bowel movements, and more. This water is finally able to create a flush-like effect and start cleaning up the cells and the traffic jam, which means the body will automatically become more efficient.

Since our body is over 70 percent water, this would be the first line of action to take in order to experience a health turnaround. Even for those who don't or won't pop pills or take supplements, this would be the simplest and most impactful nutrient to introduce. Another very attractive feature of this filter is that it produces very high alkaline water at 11.5 pH, which is not for drinking but cleaning all vegetables and fruits. In just five minutes of soaking, the water turns a pale to dark yellow! This is actually the pesticides that have been sprayed on the produce. All pesticides are oil-based; else rainwater in the fields in which they grow would wash them away. The oil base is what enables it to stick to the plants. The high-alkaline water works like an emulsifier to get the fats off effectively, and creates a visible difference. In utilizing this way, you minimize your toxic load, and food literally tastes sweeter (try eating tomatoes before and after washing to taste the difference).

If you would like to know more about the Kangen filter or how to purchase, please see the resources section at the end of the book.

Masaru Emoto, the famous Japanese professor who conducted experiments on water discovered that all conditions being equal, water has a memory: it holds the structure of the resonance it is exposed to. What this means is that if you expose the water to joyful music, it will restructure to create a beautiful crystalline pattern like a snowflake to reflect the frequency. Similarly with words of hate or anger, it will restructure to form asymmetric non-coherent patterns of dissonance.

This revelation is very important as it also proves the theory of blessing food or praying before we eat. It also means that our thoughts are restructuring physical matter! That leads us to the tangent of quantum physics, which is too large a topic for this book.

The theory of homeopathic medicine is also based on the premise that water retains a memory, thus creating medicinal values in solutions that have been diluted up to two hundred times or more.

Scientists have studied the holy water of Lourdes in France and other places where holy water phenomena or healing waters are said to occur. The common thread they found in all these spiritual waters was the fact that they had a much lower surface tension than normal water, clearly making it easier to be absorbed by the body, or more bioavailable. I would encourage you to view the entire experiment carried out by Dr. Emoto; he took photographs of the water crystals, and the pictures produced by the water are mesmerizing and a special treat for children to learn from!

If you would like to exercise a cheaper option to the Kangen filter, it won't be the same thing as creating micro cluster water, but based on Dr.

Emoto's proof, you can choose to buy an Aura Soma Water stick, that has shown to produce the most beautiful water crystals. It is a "wand" that holds very high vibrations through crystals, color, and plant essences. More in the resources section on where you can purchase it.

Dr Masaru Emoto experimented with frozen water crystals, after subjecting the water to one type of thought or picture eg: Love and gratitude, or the Beatles song 'Yesterday'. Or he labeled the water 'you disgust me.'

The results are absolutely stunning and reveal pristine sacred geometry crystals of positive thought forms and unstructured, darker forms with the negative thoughts/labels. Please see the various stunning photographs on his website for a better idea www.masaru-emoto.net/english/water-crystal.html- He also proved that such unstructured water could be just blessed or prayed upon to create the beautiful geometry again.. So our thoughts are creating us, our reality and our body (which is over 70% water anyway).

And as they say, be careful what you wish for!

Did You Know?

Bee pollen is an amazing super food with all nutrients: amino acids, vitamins, minerals, enzymes, and antioxidants, which make it one of the most preferred foods that athletes use for increased endurance and stamina.

It was a pleasure meeting Sheeba! She is so cheerful and vivacious!
I have been diabetic since 15 years and have been on insulin for
the last 2 years. My biggest worry was that despite good eating
habits and a healthy lifestyle, my sugar levels were increasing and

so was my insulin dosage. I tried different remedies & therapies but nothing worked and this often left me feeling frustrated and depressed.

Sheeba checked my blood test and medical records and made a detox plan and put me on supplements for six weeks.I felt no weakness following the restricted diet and within three weeks my insulin dosage had to be reduced by 6 units. After 2 months, my sugar levels were lower, my tummy fat reduced and the pigmentation on my cheeks disappeared!All my aches and pain have vanished and I feel twenty years younger!

Thank you Sheeba! God Bless!

R.A, Female, 71yrs

CHAPTER 5

EVERYDAY POISON

I know I have been talking a lot about our exposure to external toxins, but there is one poison we all willingly love to take.

Let's do this simple exercise for ourselves or for our loved ones.

We are going to count the number of teaspoons of sugar we are consuming in a day. Don't consume any? You will be shocked...

Let's just take breakfast:

Bowl of cereal: up to 35 g of sugar in the children's cereals=7 tsp of sugar

Orange juice: 1.5 tsp/glass (even those with no sugar added)

Cup of coffee: 1 tsp sugar

Snack: fruit yogurt (store bought) 15 g of sugar=3 tsp (in the little single cup!)

Lunch:

Veggies, noodles, chicken, and a glass of lemon lime juice with honey=1 tsp sugar (honey is a sweetener)

Snack: fruit and nut bar: up to 7-10 g sugar=1.5 tsp sugar

Dinner:

Soup, salad, and rice with curry=no desserts=no sugar

But, even without a dessert, you have tried to choose fairly healthy at all meals, and still ended up consuming 15 teaspoons of sugar!

Sugar is a sweet poison that is now linked to cancer and other chronic conditions. Why is it such a great evil? Because it is the ultimate anti-nutrient: it tastes good but takes nutritional stores away from the body, depleting them. Sugar is also inversely proportionate to immunity—studies show that the higher a person's sugar intake, the lower the immunity and vice versa. It is also the culprit in people gaining *fat*. It is not eating fat that increases this as quickly as eating sugars. Sugar creates an increase in insulin, which in turn instructs the body to store the calories as fat. This is the one thing that mainly leads to visceral fat or the fat around the belly.

Sometimes the problem is we don't even intentionally eat sugar. It's hidden in so many foods it's shocking. I had a client who got along her garlic salt to show me—it had maltodextrin in it! This is an artificial sweetener that "enhances" flavor. High-fructose corn syrup and artificial sweeteners trick the brain—they provide the sweet taste, but no nutrients or calories, so the brain wants more (nutrients) even as it gets less. Hidden sugars are now ubiquitous, so the only way to be a smart shopper is to get educated on being able to identify ingredients and labels, e.g.: concentrated grape juice. This is technically not sugar but works just like a sweetener.

So if sugar is such a big culprit, then why do we crave it?

As hunter-gatherers during times of scarcity, there was a need to store fat in the body as the main fuel. More food and calories were welcome, as one did not know when the next meal was coming. This is still the case. Sugar is actually a greater evil than fat. *It is the increased insulin response to this food that instructs the body to store the fat.* Fats in food actually lower the insulin response. This is ironic, as a lot of people shun fats in their diet but have no qualms eating high-glycemic or sugary foods.

The food industry knows this secret and uses it to create cravings for their products. It's a great taste enhancer, so it is even in items like garlic salt! But, with it being anti-nutrient, it creates a lack in the body, which then makes it want more (nutrients), and there is a vicious cycle of craving.

Sugar is the biggest anti-nutrient that creates nutritional lack as well as an acidic pH. There are many healthier alternatives to sugar, but all to be used in moderation.

My personal favorite, which is actually beneficial to the body and even diabetics, is stevia, a natural sweetener. Beware the long ingredient list that tablet and powder versions may have. Liquids are the safest, as stevia can be very expensive. It actually has a bitter molecule attached to its very sweet molecule, which may leave an unpleasant aftertaste that so many manufacturers try to mask with other ingredients and sweeteners. There are flavored liquid versions available that work to mask the taste as well. There are other sweeteners than can be used instead of sugar, in order of preference:

1. Coconut sugar
2. Yacon Syrup
3. Date syrup
4. Whole dates
5. Dried figs
6. Brown rice syrup/ prunes
7. Manuka honey/raw honey

8.   Xylitol

9.   Palm sugar (unrefined)/molasses

10. Jaggery (unrefined)

Please note I have not mentioned agave or fruit sugars. Eating fruits is very different from the fructose sugar that is available in the market, and does not behave in the same way. Agave is an extract and may only be slightly better than white sugar—it has no nutrient value to offer like jaggery, which is high in mineral content.

Artificial sweeteners are the worst choice for adults and kids alike as they have long-term side effects that are not predictable, and large amounts are known to be carcinogenic. Best avoided, even by diabetics.

Please note that stevia is a natural sweetener and therefore cannot be patented by a company. Artificial sweeteners are patented isolated creations that spin a lot of money. Most people have heard of aspartame but not stevia for the same reason. If something is not FDA-approved, (stevia was not for many years) it does not mean it is unsafe for consumption. It simply cuts into the million-dollar industry of artificial sweeteners who were the main lobbyists against it. In fact, if you dig deeper you will find that every single artificial sweetener is toxic to humans, despite being FDA approved.

Fruit Sugars: This is another area of contention. Fruits are nature's natural desserts. But there is a difference in how it should be eaten. Too many or just a plate of fruits for a meal is a shortsighted approach. There are many "natural" foods recommended for detoxing, and solely eating fruits for all your meals is not advised. But I have found my clients who follow this don't do very well digestive wise, or even with respect to their blood test results; it simply creates imbalances, as other food groups have not been included that are essential for all body systems.

EATING VERSUS DRINKING:

Eating a fruit is very different from drinking it as a fresh juice. Eating it is a slow process that needs mastication and there is a slow release of these fruit sugars into the blood stream as digestion begins. With a juice, there is a very quick release of these sugars into the blood stream as very little digestion is required. This creates a quick sugar high that works to signal to the body to store the calories as fat. Fruit is best eaten, not drunk.

I find that those who have kids that aren't fond of eating fruits, tend to give them fruit juices, fresh or bottled. This creates greater chances of cavities and further sugar cravings. It is fine however, to sweeten a vegetable juice with some small fruit, like apple.

Most households also eat fruits as a dessert after a meal, and all over the world fruit is served as a dessert. I would recommend that fruits be eaten on their own (as a snack) or before the meal, as simple sugars eaten last tend to ferment in the gut. This can cause bloating and discomfort for some. It may not have to do with the specific fruit, just the fact that it is consumed at the end of the meal.

It goes without saying that canned fruit of any kind is best avoided, as it is no longer under the definition of "real foods."

Canned foods are dead foods that contain minimum nutrients. For example, kidney beans are naturally very high in potassium—98 percent potassium, which is a beneficial mineral for us, versus two percent sodium. But the canning process completely reverses this ratio, to 98 percent sodium and two percent potassium! Those who are recommended to stay away from salt don't even realize that there is so much hidden sodium in all canned foods.

Did You Know?

Chocolate is another high antioxidant superfood, BUT only if it's raw, stone ground, and without the typical additives and sugar. There are such raw chocolates available that create health. You can look in organic stores near you and treat yourself to healthy cacao, the Food of the Gods.

When I came to see Sheeba two years ago I had spondylosis, childhood psoriasis, food sensitivities with candida overgrowth and was also experiencing hormonal swings all by age 38. The doctors did not have a cure for any of these conditions which turned out to be a blessing. The reason why I took two years to write this testimonial is because it has been an amazing journey of healing with Sheeba, culminating in ALL my issues in effect being CURED. My childhood psoriasis was clear! I also was told be a medical intuitive that my body was much better than is has ever been. What a splendid gift! Thank you Sheeba from the bottom of my heart. I will continue to recommend you to all I know because what you do — doctors simply can't. I recommend everyone to follow her advice on all aspects with an open mind as as she has a wealth of knowledge that gets to the roots of the issues. Bless you Sheeba to continue this work.

S.B, 41yrs, consultant, Female

CHAPTER 6

WEIGHT MANAGEMENT

There are books written on this topic alone, so I am devoting a chapter to it. I find that all diets and programs are successful to some degree, but the crux of it is in maintaining the weight loss. I have personal trainers who ask me why their clients who watch what they eat and train with them regularly don't shed even an ounce of weight. This directly points to sluggish metabolism, but should also ring alarm bells in those individuals: if something is not working, then the engine is faulty. Get it checked, like you would your car.

First, those who tend to put on weight on a holiday and tend to lose once they watch their diet or exercise, know that it is a losing battle as eventually you will put on a little each year in this manner, lose it all and gain it all at some point. I advise such people to get a comprehensive blood test done and get a professional to pinpoint areas of metabolism to figure out why it is so sluggish, and study subclinical parameters in the blood. I will discuss assessments in another chapter in detail, but investigative work is required.

The correct principle of weight loss to keep in mind is *not* how much weight you have lost, but how much body fat and visceral fat (fat around the organs) have decreased while maintaining or increasing muscle mass.

Muscle mass is our burning engine that helps burn calories even when we sleep or sit. This at no point in time should be compromised, which is often what happens when people go on a low-calorie diet, fast, or fall sick and suddenly lose weight. It also creates sagging and a haggard look. Visceral fat is the fat around the organs, it's the main culprit in creating disease, and is also a disease multiplier (increases complications and risk criteria). This fat and muscle mass can be measured using a galvanic current body scanner in the weighing machine itself.

Visceral fat is hard to lose; even among joggers and marathon runners, you may see they still sport a small paunch. There are some who are willing to try liposuction to remove those stubborn fats, only to die on the surgery table, as it is a dangerous procedure. In fact, in almost every marathon you hear of young or fit individuals collapsing and dying. This is the difference I would like to highlight: being seemingly fit does not equate to being healthy.

At this juncture, I would like to mention glycemic index and glycemic-loaded diets. Most people are familiar with high-glycemic foods like watermelon. They are sweet, and the higher the glycemic index of a food, the more reason to avoid them as it can be an indicator of quick sugar in the blood stream. But it isn't as simple as that. Watermelon is higher in the glycemic index than chocolate. So is it better to eat chocolate? Two things to watch out for here: amount or quantity definitely matters, and nutrients always need to matter. This is where glycemic load comes in, where quantity of the food is taken into account along with glycemic index. The rule is not to exceed over GL 40 per meal. This helps to reduce or maintain weight. You can find the glycemic load of foods online. So in this case, a small piece of chocolate can compare to a big bowl of watermelon. This would be a little more accurate reflection of how to eat.

It also allows one to eat what you want in restricted, sensible portions.

After having done many diets and maybe even losing a certain chunk of weight, some people reach a plateau and just aren't able to lose any more. For such people, there is a fantastic solution.

HCg and HA2CG Homeopathic Weight Management Diet:

The HCg diet started over 25 years ago, and was fine-tuned by Dr. Simeons. HCg stands for human chorionic gonadotropin, a hormone that is produced in large amounts in pregnant women. It helps to mobilize fat stores to be made available to the fetus and growing mother. It is this hormone that was injected in morbidly obese patients who were fed low-calorie, no-fat diets during that time with astonishing results. Despite the low-calorie diet, not a single patient lost any muscle mass, but kept losing abnormal fat stores, especially visceral fat, or the fat around the organs. They retained or gained muscle mass during the entire program. Weight loss was rapid, but without the haggard look—each one looked toned fitter, and younger.

Here is where I know some of you may be jumping at the fact that I am recommending a ridiculous, low-calorie diet that sounds more like a crash diet. How can that improve health? I have personally seen over 400 clients who have done this very diet with me with the intention of weight loss, but instead what they got was life-changing: a complete health transformation.

Some key points to highlight here:

» All regular low-calorie diets will lead to muscle mass loss, including fasting. During the HCG diet you will not lose any muscle mass, but instead gain it. This is NOT a regular low-calorie diet.

» It helps mobilize abnormal fat stores including the visceral fat around the organs. It is important, as this is the main culprit and disease multiplier: the higher your organ fats, the higher your disease(s) factor, including hormonal issues.

» If you are using the correct HCG (without any hormone derivatives), then it actually helps to balance hormones, instead of the other way around.

» For those who have done it and found success, you know it works. But for those who have done it and have regained the weight, you need to examine why. That's why I always recommend doing a blood test before embarking on any weight loss program; so you can identify problem areas or fill in nutrient gaps (e.g., low iron levels or having a fatty liver). Such issues will slow down your metabolism tremendously if not addressed. Have you addressed low iron issues through weight loss? Certainly not. You will still feel fatigue, maybe even worse after the diet. That doesn't have anything to do with the diet. But this is what creates negative experiences and misinformation on the Internet.

» Since toxins are stored in your fat cells, especially the visceral fat, during the program there are a lot of toxins being released. It is essential to support all the detoxification systems during the program. Most herbs interfere with the HCG program, so some homeopathically based detox support is required. This will also prevent recirculation of toxins in your system and improve overall health at the same time.

» Constipation can be a challenge for some on the program, so make sure you are taking some bowel support to prevent recirculation of toxins.

» Many reputed integrated doctors offer this program. I know many have successfully done the DIY approach, but for permanent and improved health, and for reasons listed above, please do seek a professional who can look into all the above criteria.

» A galvanic weighing scale that measures muscle mass, body fat percent, and visceral fat would be very useful, as this helps to monitor if you are moving in the right direction.

» The HCG diet is a double-edged sword: if done correctly, the results are spectacular, if not, you can end up putting on weight instead. It is important to be sure about the exact protocols.

» The right products are also key for best results and health—there are HCG drops available in Wal-Mart for about 20 U.S. dollars. Not all products are created equal, so use caution.

Another overlooked issue is clients who come to me with goals like "get rid of diabetes." I know this to be possible, but somehow there is a disconnect between the client's intentions and goals. When I recommend what they can do to reach their goal, offering bite-sized portions of "doables" at a time, they back out and mumble an apology, but at this point they only want some input to change their diet.

I had a male client who came to me with these exact goals and health concerns. I looked at his blood test and figured that he was a smoker. He was an ex-smoker who had quit a few years ago. He was surprised I found out from the blood tests, as he had not mentioned this in his health questionnaire. I frankly told him that his body was still nutritionally deficient from years of smoking, and full of toxins that needed to be cleared up—whether he did it slowly or with the HCG diet was up to him.

The client refused to take any supplements despite his results showing the deficiencies. He simply wanted a diet to follow for his diabetic condition. At times this is very frustrating for me as a health-care practitioner, as I know they can be helped, but you can only help those who choose to help themselves. There is a disconnect with intention and their achievable goals.

Also, for many clients, all decisions are from fear-based thinking. They can take drugs prescribed by doctors, with a multitude of side effects, but swallowing a supplement is, in their minds, too much of a stretch. All such clients have a slim chance of really improving their health—managing their health concerns, yes, but not improving them.

It is important that you examine your intentions, actions, and reasons: some people prefer their diseased state, as they achieve negative attention with it. When you really yearn for a transformation, you will ask all the right questions and the right people will come to you.

Sorry for the deviation—examining your motives is the key to success.

Getting back to the diet: **HA2CG miracle.**

There are many variations to the HCG diet, and not everyone wants to take injections or use hormones, as we don't know the long-term consequences of such use.

The one I use and recommend to overweight patients is practitioner-grade, homeopathic, sublingual drops that are not derived from the hormone, but have amino acid sequences in there that mimic the effects of HCG, creating a similar effect with no long or short-term consequences. In fact, I do a before and after blood test with each client showing improved test results on all health parameters. There are many who do it for weight loss but find that it has helped reduce their insulin dosage, their medications, and actually cleared up some health concerns completely, especially autoimmune.

Having said that, it is not very easy for vegetarians to follow, as the food can be monotonous and the diet itself is for a minimum three weeks of no fats, specific foods only after which is three weeks of a maintenance phase where fats are allowed with a wider range of food choices. Know that the HCG diet is remarkable and works 100 percent for anyone embarking on weight loss, but is a double-edged sword: if done incorrectly, you can put on weight instead of losing. Another consideration is, since you are mobilizing fat stores, you also mobilize toxins at the same time, as most toxins are stored in fat cells. Because of this, all detoxification systems need to be supported during the diet. After the no-fat phase, the client needs to incorporate fats and all vitamins, minerals, and antioxidants, which have been depleted during the no-fat phase. Due to all the criteria, it is best to contact a professional who has experience with this diet.

WHO SHOULD EMBARK ON THIS DIET?

» Those who have tried to lose weight naturally with a sensible diet and exercise but have not seen results
» Those with very high body fat and visceral fat
» Those with hormonal and/or thyroid challenges
» Those with multiple health challenges
» Those with autoimmune challenges
» Those taking medications who want to reduce the amount taken

Other Programs that Work: If there are people who are unable to commit to something so rigid, then another weight management solution is available. I still recommend you get some baseline assessment like a blood test done, to identify nutrient highs or lows before you start any program.

This twelve-week package is available from Pharmanex, whose products are sold through network marketing. Their products are not meal replacements, and are safe for teenagers and seniors as well. They incorporate the same philosophy of decreasing body fat, while increasing muscle mass to gain sustainable and long-term results. The supplements help to reduce visceral fat, while reducing the insulin response after we eat.

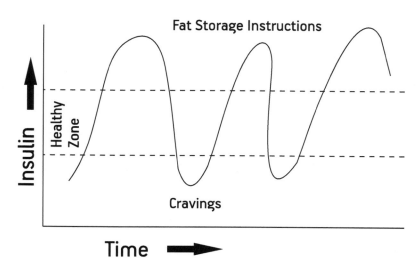

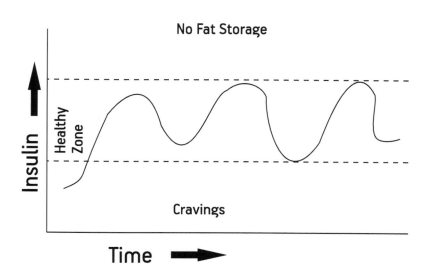

If you see this graph, you will find that after a certain point, the insulin levels instruct the body to store those calories as fat. If we are able to reduce this insulin response, we no longer store fat and instead the present fat stores are used for metabolism.

I have many clients with diabetes type I and type II who especially get very good results on this program, to the point where they can reduce other medications. There are other leaner clients who use this program to alter their body composition. I had a marathon runner who came to me whose body fat percent was already at 12 percent. He wanted to get to nine percent body fat without compromising his muscle mass, endurance, or stamina. As he was already into heavy exercise routine and watching his diet, he was skeptical when I shared this weight program with him. After doing the program, however, he came down to nine percent body fat in three weeks, with no change in body weight, as his muscle mass had increased. He also stopped getting muscle cramps, and his stamina had gone up.

When we mobilize and burn fat stores, we also mobilize toxins. So fat stores equate to toxins. We feel better as aches and pains decrease; inflammation markers also abate with loss of fat. It is a better way to detox than to cut calories or go on other fad diets.

TR90

Nuskin has a new package that is called TR90, that is the first weight-management product in the world that works on switching off our fat genes—all food-based supplements are safe, even for obese or overweight children. I have personally tried it and found it to be effective. What convinced me to try it was the solid genetic science and research behind the product.

PURIUM:

This is another network marketing brand available in the United States that has very affordable weight loss ten-day transformation plans. All their products are food-based, science-based, and mostly organic, so even if you don't know where to start with detox or supplements, or getting nutritious products, this brand wins hands-down. They have great protein powders, vegetables, and super foods. Their ten-day transformation package can be extended to suit your weight-loss needs.

THRIVE LEVEL:

This is another brand that delivers what it promises. It has a very simple program of taking a micro-ionized multi-nutrient protein-based shake, a supplement formulated for men and women and their DFT (Derma Fusion Technology) patches, which are stickers applied to the skin for 24 hours. The nutrients enter transdermally—which is a new technology that makes the ingredients 100 percent bioavailable, as it bypasses the digestive system. This means less swallowing of supplements, with more effectiveness. Their program is for eight weeks, to create sustainable weight loss and improve energy.

DIFFERENT DIETS:

They all work to some degree, but the principle to a good program should always be to verify that you are losing body fat, not muscle mass. At any point in time, you should not be feeling tired, hungry, or just worse off.

BLOOD TYPE DIET:

This diet, however, is not considered a diet for weight loss. This is a diet that advises you how to eat based on your blood type (A, B, or O). What the crux of this diet is, is that it removes inflammation-causing foods that react to your blood type, thus enhancing overall health and wellbeing. It is supposed to be a diet you follow for life. It has helped many to turn around their health, but again, for many it may not be practical.

KETOGENIC DIET:

This diet stays away from all grains and sugars and is a high fat diet with 50-70% calories coming from good fats. The HA2CG is also a Ketogenic diet. Such diets are the most anti-inflammatory and immune supporting.

Natural cancer institutes all over the world are adopting this diet for all cancer and auto-immune patients. By reducing the insulin response in the body, the infections can't feed off the sugars.

GLYCEMIC LOAD DIET:

This is another great way to lose or maintain your weight without too much fuss. We have all heard of glycemic index of foods. This refers to how fast the sugar in your blood would rise after eating. Glycemic load, however, refers to the quantity of the respective food eaten.

For example, you can eat an entire chocolate bar, which would create a massive sugar surge, or you could have a small square of the chocolate, which would create a smaller spike in blood sugar. Similarly, the quantity of what you eat is very important in maintaining a sugar balance in the body. Scientists found that the magic number was a glycemic load of 40. It helped to either lose or maintain the same weight, depending on what effect was desired.

That way, you don't have to deprive yourself of all the things you love, just eat in moderation. There are diet books available with recipes and their GL number. Going by glycemic load is a smarter way to eat.

TURNING AROUND HEALTH:

» To turn around health, the first step is to eliminate refined foods. This is a must.

» Then, you can eliminate all types of sugar, natural and manmade (not fruits).

» The next step could be to eliminate all wheat and dairy foods.

» Incorporate more fresh vegetables and green leafy juices—as many as you can. Even adding super green powders to this will enhance the nutrient value. Making tasty smoothies is a great way to enjoy this.

» Move to a more plant-based diet.

» Start replacing your "drinks" with pure water and herbal teas.

Tip: If you are trying to lose weight, then your mental approach needs to be changed. Think of yourself *donating* your weight. When you lose something, automatically there is a mentality to find it. When you donate, you feel good, as you have given for a good cause, without ever expecting it back. This frame of mind sets you up for permanent success.

NOTE: For children who are overweight, replacing sugary foods with healthier options and working towards a Glycemic Load 40 (GL40) may be the best way.

Another point to note is that many teenagers have little tummies still sticking out! If that is the case, they need to cut sugars but also do some gentle homeopathic cleanse/detoxification drops that clear out accumulated toxins. When you eat junk foods and drinks, there are multiple levels of toxicity that the body accumulates, and typically this will be stored in the visceral fat or tummy area, even for young children. This reflects high toxicity and extremely poor food choices as well as low nutrient levels in the body.

WEIGHT GAIN

This can be a little harder than losing weight! People who have trouble gaining weight do need to do the investigative work with assessments and blood tests. Most suffer from compromised digestive systems, a leaky gut, candida (yeast/fungus) overgrowth, poor detoxification, possibly high toxic-load, low-protein stores, and multiple food allergies. All these issues can exist simultaneously, so they need to be treated systematically in phases. I will be mentioning each of these in more detail in later chapters. Overweight people can have exactly the same issues; the only difference is how the body processes this information, e.g. creating excess or lack. People trying to put on weight may be surprised to know that a gallbladder cleanse and some detoxification is going to help them. I have clients who think because they are thin, they are exempt from doing any cleanses and such, as it is generally directed at people wanting to lose weight.

Detoxification done gently is recommended, while working on building the body at the same time, through the right nutrients. For those struggling with weight gain or loss, there is usually also a lack of self-love. The primary focus should be on instilling this. Self-love is very important for those who are bulimic or anorexic.

Instilling self-love: This is a very simple technique and can be done anywhere, anytime. Starting with your head and moving down, or vice versa, you can either touch the specific part of the body or do it mentally, and state "I love my eyes, my beautiful eyes. I am grateful and thankful for these eyes. Bless these eyes," and so on, until you are done with your entire body. This could take all of five minutes or 20 minutes, depending how much time you want to spend on yourself. I have clients who tell me they don't really believe what they are saying—and that's fine. You don't need to believe you love yourself. Just stating it and going through the process everyday will change that. It's *especially* important for those who don't believe it to do it, as they have negative body images. As you start doing this exercise, don't be surprised if you have tears—this is good. It is an emotional washing or detoxification of negative imprints that happen, and that is what we want.

Did You Know?

HIIT or high-intensity-interval training, which involves two minutes of normal paced activity, like walking, with 30 second bursts of speed (making it a jog) for six cycles, which is less than 20 minutes, is far more effective at burning fat as compared to a one hour workout? So exercise smart, not hard.

I've had Polycystic Ovarian Syndrom since I was a teenager and as a result was diagnosed with Insulin Resistance after my first pregnancy 16 years ago.

Over the years, managing my weight had become a daily struggle even with regular exercise and watching my diet. Over the last 2 years I'd put on 10 kgs. This is when I decided to consult Sheeba who recommended I start on the HCG diet program. I started with 3 weeks and decided to extend for another 3 as I saw and felt the amazing results I was getting in my body. I was loosing weight at the right places (belly fat, and thighs), my body fat was going down, but my muscle mass was also building. More than

than, I was feeling good and energised, contrary to the numerous diets I'd tried in the past.

My weekly visit to Sheeba was so motivating as I could see the weight and measurements improving every time. The diet is strict but still was not difficult to follow as I was not hungry at all.

I am now on maintenance and feel that the food I eat this suits me totally. I continue to maintain and even loose weight. I feel in control again. I finally feel confident about my body but mostly I feel good and when I eat with no bloating or digestion difficulties.

I was on Metformin (diabetes control medication) before starting the program and I am off now. I feel my sugar level is under control and I have no cravings or energy fluctuation. I am waiting for a few more weeks before I go for a total check up and check my insulin resistance status and other blood readings.

I am very grateful for Sheeba to have guided me through this journey of transforming my health and my body!"

Valerie M. 44yrs

CHAPTER 7

THE DIGESTIVE SYSTEM: GREAT WALL OF CHINA AND SECOND BRAIN

The digestive system is the most complex and fascinating system in the body. This system is supported by all other systems, creating a domino effect on health.

At this point there is a sequence of digestion that needs to be understood:

Mouth: Chews food, and saliva releases amylase enzymes to start the carbohydrate digestion process.

Stomach: Hydrochloric acid from the stomach creates a highly acidic pH, which is conducive for protein breakdown, and promotes mineral absorption. Intrinsic factor secretion helps to absorb vitamin B12.

Small Intestine: This is home to two-thirds of the immune system, and is the largest part of the digestive system. When spread out, it has the surface area of an entire football field. The little projections or microvilli in the intestine create multiple folds, which help expose the food to the maximum area for complete digestion and absorption. Chronic exposure to inflammatory agents can cause damage to the intestinal lining, creating a leaky gut.

Large Intestine: Gut floras synthesize vitamins and further breakdown non-digestible carbohydrates. Sodium and water is reabsorbed at this point, and remains are eliminated.

The digestive center is also a prominent part of the immune system, comprising of 70 percent of immune protection. This alone gives it the privileged platform of being the center of attention and first area of investigation for all traditional systems of medicine. They all believe that 99 percent of diseases stem from the gut.

At this point, pH needs to be well understood. The blood pH needs to be kept at a slightly alkaline pH of 7.3. It is imperative for the body to maintain this pH, in order to prevent any critical conditions like shock, etc.

The stomach pH needs to be very acidic (pH 1 to 4), in order to ensure protein digestion, absorption of minerals, and B vitamins. The small intestines enzymatically create an alkaline pH to neutralize the acidic pH from the stomach. It also has the main function of absorbing nutrients and then passing on the remains to the large intestine for further absorption and clearing.

Most people's digestive tracts aren't working optimally, so it's no surprise when kids complain of tummy aches and adults feel bloated.

The Second Brain: Gut instinct. When it comes to your mood, decisions, and behaviors, it's not just your brain doing all the work. The body contains a separate nervous system that comprises of 5,000,000 neurons—in your GUT! This unique system is called the Enteric Nervous System, also dubbed the "Second Brain." It shares some common features with the brain–did you know that your gut produces over 40 different neurotransmitters? One of which is serotonin, a well-known neurotransmitter that improves mood and sleep. Ninety-five percent of serotonin is produced in the gut. So if you are an emotional eater, you know why. The health of your gut is important for better health and mood. Depending on what you eat, your behavior, decisions, and personality change! This is dramatically obvious in children with high food sensitivities and autism.

Leaky Gut Syndrome: This is when the intestinal tract absorbs things it otherwise wouldn't, while undigested food particles move out, which are not recognized by the immune system. Toxins and bacteria normally barricaded by the Great Wall are now allowed entry. The immune system is compromised, initiating a low-grade inflammatory response, where symptoms are vast. Pathogenic microbes impair immunity, cause chronic infections, and release toxic compounds through their own life cycle, causing further distress and burden on our immune systems, which is also known as Dysbiosis. This creates mineral imbalances, leading to deficiencies like low iron, low zinc, etc. that can further choke up the liver detoxification systems, increasing toxin build-up.

Symptoms of leaky gut can range from:

» IBS

» Crohn's/Colitis

» Dermatitis, eczema, hives, skin rashes, acne

» Insulin insensitivity

- » PCOS
- » Asthma, wheezing, runny nose
- » Headaches
- » Weight gain
- » Chronic fatigue/fibromyalgia
- » Autoimmune diseases
- » Joint pains
- » Depression, anxiety, mental fog
- » Adrenal fatigue
- » Systemic inflammation

OVER ACID OR UNDER ACID?

Doctors tell their patients that they have reflux due to over acidity. This is technically correct, but not the entire picture. Ninety percent of individuals have low stomach acid. If there were high stomach acid, it would help to break down food and help absorb nutrients and cause less digestive problems. Those with truly high acid have an overproduction of acid and can use herbs that reduce this acid burn.

Most who think they have high acid: think again. The typical scenario is due to low stomach acid: the food lies in the stomach, the stomach tries to produce acid for digestion, but meanwhile the food moves along the intestines for further digestion. But since the initial proteins have not digested due to lack of stomach acid, there is poor digestion, heavy burden on the intestines, and fermentation of food, leading to bloatedness and unease, lack of appetite, and so on. Meanwhile, the stomach still hasn't stopped trying to produce acid, and when there is no food in the stomach, there are sudden bursts of acid production that have happened at the wrong time, creating acid burps and reflux.

Everyone with over acid or under acid production, including seemingly normal people and kids, will find that they have less trouble when they eat every two and a half to three hours. It may not be a meal, but a small snack like a small fruit and some nuts.

Adding a teaspoon of apple cider vinegar (dilute as required) before each of your main meals can help improve stomach pH and assist in balance.

But it doesn't solve the issue of the low stomach-acid production. There are many reasons for this, the primary one being stress or nervousness that switches off the digestive tract in order to conserve energy (a lot of energy goes into digesting food!). That's why you have the saying, "butterflies in my stomach," as a sign of nervousness. The other primary reason is when there is a direct interference with the stomach acid production in some manner. Our very old amalgam mercury fillings are major culprits, however, it could also be tobacco intake or smoking. I will discuss this in the next chapter, dealing with everyday toxins that directly effect health.

When the stomach pH is not as acidic as it should be (pH one to four), then the digestive system is topsy-turvy. The acidic pH protects and prevents any bacteria and pathogens from surviving. But when the pH is not what it should be, it propagates bacteria (*H. Pylori* is common). Mlabsorption starting in the stomach carries all the way down into the gut, leading to fermentation. This starts to create an acidic environment in the blood. Confusing, but simplistically put, if the body's ability to absorb nutrients that assist in detoxifying the body is compromised, then what builds up is acid or toxins. So, blood pH becomes more acidic than its usual 7.3 pH.

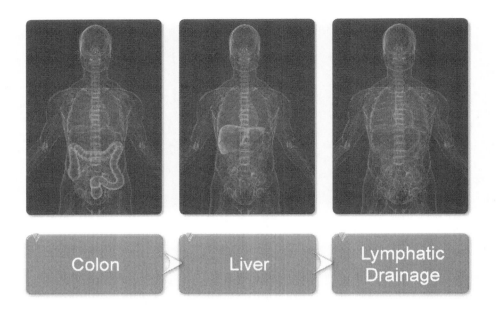

This sets up a chain reaction creating multiple health issues. Once minerals are low, the body's protective mucus lining around the gut and stomach wears thin, creating gaps that acid can eat into, causing ulcers.

WHAT YOU CAN DO:

You can replace your metal fillings with ceramic ones, and take apple cider vinegar to directly improve stomach pH levels. Dilute as necessary before meals. Mineral and amino acid stores need to be restored, so trace minerals and other nutrients are very important for this.

You do need to work on a detox that suits your body, so working with a healthcare practitioner is essential.

Antibiotics: What is the relevance of antibiotics in digestion? Pretty much everything. Nowadays, the use and misuse of antibiotics is rampant. Everyone is given varying doses of antibiotics. Even I was misled into taking antibiotics, when my doctor diagnosed that my cough was viral!

First, antibiotics kill bacteria, not any other type of pathogen. The way they work is to destroy the cell wall of the bacteria, essentially killing it. Antibiotics will kill *all* bacteria, good and bad.

Now let's backtrack a bit. The human adult body has over four pounds of bacteria in our system at any given time. However, we also have a finely balanced ratio of viruses, good and bad bacteria, yeast, parasites, and sometimes fungus in our bodies. It sounds gross, but they live together in equilibrium, where one microorganism fights for space against the other, and prevents the other from overgrowing.

Anything that tips the scale in favor of one over the other is the clear winner. This happens when antibiotics are introduced into the system. They kill off all bacteria, creating a huge "space" for the other organisms that are not affected by the antibiotic. There is no vacuum in nature, so this space is very readily filled up by overgrowth of the friendly yeast in our gut called Candida.

Meanwhile, with frequent use of antibiotics, the intestinal lining (the Great wall of China), which typically renews and repairs itself every three days, has a harder time to do so. This creates "gaps" or permeable areas in the intestinal wall, which compromise gut integrity. This means that things (undigested food matter) that should remain in the gut start to move out, and infections and pathogens that should stay out have a chance to move in, thus compromising the immune system. This creates **food allergy** patterns that progressively increase while depressing the immune system. This issue is termed as a permeable gut or a "leaky gut" by natural health-care practitioners.

What this means to an individual with a leaky gut, is that there is undigested food moving out that is not recognized by the immune system, which instead identifies it as a pathogen and thus attacks it. This creates a cascading immune response, producing inflammation, irritation, mucus, and allergy patterns.

Candida overgrowth: Known to some and experienced by many, Candida overgrowth eludes medical doctors completely. The lifecycle of yeast is such that it grows, feeding on fermented foods and carbohydrates, creating further fermentation in the gut. The growth of yeast takes on a fungal form and in their life cycle, the fungus releases over 75 different mycotoxins in the gut *everyday*, creating a massive and sudden onslaught of toxic load. This is like constantly battering your immune system and detoxification systems as well.

What happens to the body? The mycotoxins also weaken the Great Wall. As immune systems weaken, recurring minor or major illnesses can become regular phenomena. It accelerates a leaky gut, as there is more damage being done to the digestive tract than it has the time to repair and renew. The leaky gut further increases losses of nutrients and also increases food allergies. Candida further encourages the growth of bad bacteria, so flare up of fungal or bacterial infections are common.

Other issues experienced could be:

1. All skin conditions, including: psoriasis, eczema, urticaria, and fungal nails and skin.

2. Digestive issues from minor to major: food allergies, indigestion, bloating, etc.

3. Poor growth, food absorption, recurring stomach pain

4. Headaches, migraines, general inflammation

5. Hormonal imbalances, mood swings

6. May cause deeper immune weakness leading to mycoplasma, herpes, etc.

7. Sinusitis, nasal congestion, post-nasal drip

8. Mental fog, unclear thinking

9. Depression, anxiety

10. Weight gain or weight loss

11. Irritable Bowel Syndrome

12. Recurring infections like urinary tract or thrush

13. Lymph congestion, swelling

14. Upper and lower respiratory-tract chronic issues

15. Recurring illnesses like herpes and other infections

16. Cravings for sugary or salty foods

17. Hypoglycemia or sudden drop in blood sugar levels

18. Progressive food allergies; leaky gut

Doctors do not even recognize this as a health concern or disease they need to look into. So it is never investigated and thus many a time, symptoms are termed "idiopathic" (meaning: I don't know how it came to be) or the patient is referred to a specialist. And the story goes on...

I was told by my medical doctors that nothing could be done about my fatty liver, definitely not reverse it, and that I should always avoid fatty foods due to that. I went to Sheeba for weight loss, and instead, to my amazement, she rightly said that if we give the body what it needs, it can repair itself – and after the program with her, I felt much better, but my blood test results reflected that in black and white – My liver enzymes were within normal range! That was the gift of health for me and I am very grateful to Sheeba for transforming my weight and health " ...

Joy C – Male, 38 yrs, Consultant

CHAPTER 8

RESTORING GUT EQUILIBRIUM

All good nutrition books will guide you on four fundamental principles of restoring gut balance. The key is using the right supplements that are most effective and least "disturbing" to our bodies. Gentler is better than hard core here. I come across many clients who are fans of detoxing every six months and try different methods to work "deeper" on themselves. These people end up with diarrhea, feel ill, lose muscle mass, and even go hypoglycemic to the point of fainting.

I am not keen on this approach, as these detoxes do not have to torture the body in any way and doing it wrong can literally poison you and make things worse.

Sometimes just choosing to eliminate sugar can be a detox. Drinking more water can assist in the process, and tweaking it to a whole foods diet can also work as a detox. To create a healthier you, please refrain from DIY approaches. I do recommend taking key supplements that support the body's detoxification pathways without making you feel like crap. For children who need to detoxify, I always recommend the state-of-the-art 21st century homeopathic range from Deseret Biologicals. These are so gentle yet work very deep, where most botanicals cannot even reach. They are safe for all ages and appropriate for adults as well. In fact, I get the best results with these homeopathies than all past supplements I have used for detoxing.

Under the care of a health practitioner, there is a protocol that they would need to follow, called the four golden R's:

The Four R's:

REMOVE:

» Pathogens (the bad guys): Identifying this may be a nightmare. Many parasites go undetected, so it is important to make sure you choose the right assessment(s). Mycoplasma is a tricky one too, but normally a blood test will pick it up.

» Foods creating inflammation or triggers—normally the practitioner will provide a doable detox diet that can be for 14 to 21 days. For some with serious or chronic issues, even a food allergy assessment may be warranted here.

» Toxins (getting to the source of toxicity, e.g., amalgam fillings): this is key if you wish to see permanent results.

» Desensitizing to food allergies and triggers. This can be done by going to a NAET (Namboodiripad Allergy Elimination Test) practitioner, or by using the Deseret Biologicals (see appendix) food sensitivity kits. This step is not specific to all, only those who have serious leaky gut issues, as determined by your practitioner.

REPLACE:

» Digestive support with either digestive enzymes or Betaine HCl to improve stomach acid digestion.

» Improve gastric secretions and optimize stomach pH.

REPAIR:

» Soothe, build, and repair gut lining and intestinal wall—the L glutamine, aloe vera, slippery elm, marshmallow root, and glucosamine work in combination to help with this repair work. Normally this is introduced after the detox or Phase One.

RE-INOCULATE:

» With good gut bacteria. Not just any probiotic will do. Ninety percent or more of the probiotics on the shelf today have been found to have very little or no real impact in turning around gut health. Make sure it is a good one that does make the difference. I personally prefer food based fermented probiotics like Dr. Xeniji, Microbiomax, or Ohhira probiotics (see appendix for product details). This can be taken from the start of the detox program.

I came to Sheeba to address my 10 yr old daughter's digestive problems. She was extremely underweight, had frequent tummy aches and hardly eats much. Sheeba recommended that she undergoes a complete food desensitization program to heal her digesive issues. My daughter has a twin borther who is autistic. Sheeba suggested that he can also follow the same treatment protocol. I had tried bio-medical and GCFC before for my son without much improvement. It has now been 3 months into the treatment and I have begun to see trmendous improvement in both my children. My daughter's tummy ache is almost non existent now and her appetite has imporved dramatically. She is now beginning to to put on weight. My son's behaviour has changed tremendously and is something that I had not seen with any other treatment to date. He is much better eye contact, smiling more and his level of understanding has increased. Sheeba's approach to healing the body's natural healing process has actually helped both my children. My children are well on the path to recovery and I am very excited with the progress so far. I am very greatful to Sheeba for this transformation in their health and for all the help and guidance."

G.S, 40, Homemaker

CHAPTER 9

SOURCE OF ALL ILLNESS

An experiment was conducted many years ago using cell tissues from a chicken. The experiment was simple: every day the solution had to be changed with a new one and then monitored to see how long it would last in a clean environment. This went on for years, with the solution in the petri dish with the living cells being changed every day of every year, for 56 years. The cells had already outlived the regular age of a chicken.

One day, the person in charge forgot to change the solution, and the next day the cells had all but died.

What this experiment intended to prove was how long cells can survive if there is no toxicity, and if they are given daily nutrients. The results were cut short, but the trial was long enough to reveal that cells can far outlive the general cap on aging if the conditions are right. That is why the actual calculated biological age of a human's life span is 120 years, which people have lived up to, albeit a handful.

Our very thoughts can change the structure and outcome of cellular processes, but Dr. Bruce Lipton best elaborates that in one of my favorite books, *The Biology of Belief*.

Our thoughts and beliefs create patterns and can be a source of mental and emotional toxicity. I would like to mention some common physical toxicity that creates chronic stress in the body, eventually leading to all disease.

Mercury amalgam fillings: This metal filling was used as a cheaper substitute for gold. Each amalgam filling has over 50 percent mercury in it, along with other metals. These fillings have now been banned in countries like Canada and Europe. According to the WHO, even an atom of mercury is considered toxic, whether you ingest it, inhale it, or permanently sport it in your mouth. Dentists are in denial that they have seen any harm come of it. That's because patients come to them for their teeth, not for their health. There are many articles written on this all over the Internet. To me it's simple. If mercury is considered one of the most powerful neurotoxins (it can fuddle your brain), then do you want it permanently in your mouth? You need to become a conscious consumer and choose ceramic or gold if need be.

Each tooth, like foot reflexology, reflects and connects to different organs and meridian pathways. Depending on which tooth you have the filling in, that organ and system will systematically get a drip-drip of poison.

I do agree that each filling should have a small amount of mercury. But imagine a tap that has a leak and water drips down. This drip is not going to fill a bucket overnight. But over a period of time, the bucket will overflow!

Similarly, the mercury creates a slow, insidious poison that jams up all detoxification systems, and creates a huge toxic burden in each cell.

This poison does not show up in a typical blood test report; the body has to work smart. Instead of moving around in the blood, which actually carries precious nutrients to cells, the body sequesters these neurotoxins into the least metabolically active cells so as not to interfere with everyday cellular metabolism—these are your fat cells, especially the fat around the organs or visceral fat. But fat is in the brain tissue and can also overlap into muscles. In the brain it interferes and causes depression, Parkinson's, Alzheimer's, and other neurologically related diseases.

People who try to lose weight (especially the paunch!) find that is the last or hardest to lose despite rigorous exercise and diet. Those who lose weight but retain amalgam fillings find that their battle with weight loss is never-ending, as eventually body fat creeps back with a vengeance. This is because the body needs the fat as a buffer or cushion for the toxins, and unless the source of these toxins is removed, body fat will never reduce to optimal levels. It's a simple safety mechanism of your body trying to protect your organs against the toxins.

It is not easy to get rid of heavy metal toxicity like mercury, and requires specific nutrients that bypass the digestive system either via IV drip or via anal suppositories. This would need practitioner guidance.

If you had mercury fillings in the past but not anymore, you still need to do a complete heavy metal cleanse, so please do contact a practitioner who is knowledgeable about this.

So far we have spoken of mercury. When we have other metals placed in our body— like a copper IUD—know that they also create adverse reactions. Titanium plates, etc., all create micro-galvanic currents (we have natural electrolytes that conduct a charge in our bodies) that disrupt meridian and energy flow. There are times when it cannot be avoided, but do inquire if there are ceramic versions or newer types out in the market that may be safer.

I had a client well into her forties who was on a weight-management program with me. She diligently did her blood tests and what came up for her was heavy metal toxicity. We went through her life and couldn't really figure out where it was coming from in such a big way. She didn't have any amalgam fillings, so even that was ruled out. I make it a point to physically check my clients' teeth, as they tend to forget they actually have any!

The following week when she was back, she realized she had amalgam fillings as a teenager and got them removed and replaced in her earlier years. She had called her mum to verify that! Please note that composite or ceramic is nontoxic, but even if you replaced your amalgam years ago, you still have the old mercury creating toxicity in your system.

Another client had toxicity show up as a mystery. She had hormonal issues, candida, leaky gut, migraines, depression, and more. I was sure there was heavy-metal toxicity involved, but couldn't put my finger on it. Towards the end of the consult she just mentioned she had an IUD "if that counted". Of course! Copper is not a heavy metal, so she didn't think to mention it. The copper was depleting zinc stores and creating most of the issues that she was experiencing. It even causes aggression. So if there are men reading this, there is a reason your wife is not what she used to be! Even contraceptive pills create a similar environment, as they increase copper stores in the body. Another client had mercury show up—this client was ten years old! He had no mercury fillings. How did he get that much mercury in his system to show up in a hair mineral analysis?

Both parents had multiple amalgam fillings! So yes, unfortunately, we pass our toxins on to the growing fetus. This would also explain how babies who drink breast milk develop eczema and such—no food allergies obviously, but because toxicities have passed on from the mother to the child, and a baby is extremely sensitive to them; even in small amounts they are dangerous, as the immune system has not really kicked in.

Drinking water is another very big source of pollutants and heavy metals, including some metals like uranium and tungsten. Clean water is not only an issue in third-world countries, but the first-world countries like the United States have hormone disruptors in tap water to boot, along with fluoride.

Fluoride is in most countries' waters. It is another controversy, but again, the logic is simple. Fluoride and chlorine both displace iodine in nature. Which means, wherever there is fluoride or chlorine, iodine will not coexist. This works exactly the same in the body.

I could write an entire book on iodine, but fortunately, one has already been written by Dr. David Brownstein (*Iodine, why you need it and why you can't live without it*).

This title tells you everything. Iodine is the only mineral (out of 80) that is required for hormones, immunity, metabolism, detoxification, liver, heart, brain health, and more. We normally don't replenish our stores of iodine, as it is found only in sea vegetables and seaweed—another hint as to why Japanese are one of the longest-living humans on the planet.

In more simplistic terms, daily fluoride causes loss of metabolism and generally reduces brain alertness and function. We are creating dumber nations. Even dentists use a fluoride rinse for teeth. Please ensure you avoid this or switch to a bio dentist in your area.

Since water is the most basic nutrient, invest in a restructured water system for your entire family. Do take an iodine supplement as well to maintain optimal levels.

Other ingestible sources of metal can come from an unexpected source: your daily supplements! So beware, as your fish oils or shark fin cartilage supplement can be an everyday source. You need to make sure your supplements are clean, and it's better to take advice from a professional than self-supplement for this reason.

Copper water pipes are commonly used, and even when you're just bathing in water that has heavy metals in it, the metals are very quickly absorbed transdermally, so there is no escape there. Excess amounts of copper have been shown to lead to Alzheimer's and neurodegenerative diseases. There is a whole list of what each heavy metal does to the body in the long run. You may just have some aches and muscle pains, and these can gradually become a chronic disease. Your body is constantly sending you warning signals; so don't take it as a part of aging, but an accumulation of toxicity. That is why detoxification of some kind is featured in all the old religions as a way to cleanse. This is essential for everyone, religious or not. Please read the chapter on heavy metal chelation to learn more on how to clear these toxicities from your system.

So far we have only spoken of metal toxicity. There are myriad chemical toxicities that we are exposed to, and willingly expose ourselves to as well (like perfume, body care lotions, etc.). So how does one get rid of chemical toxicities? Please see the chapter dedicated to cleansing for more details. Homeopathic remedies that are related to specific chemical toxicities (like petrochemicals for instance) created by Deseret Biologicals are an easy way to detoxify it out of your system, especially if you have a child who cannot do cleansing.

I came to Sheeba on a friend's recommendation, as I had been beset with digestive problems and recurring infections for more than a year. I was tired of taking medication that addressed only symptoms, but not the root of my problems, so I decided to give a more holistic approach a try. Sheeba took the time to go through the results of various health reports with me in detail, which helped me to understand the systemic issues behind the symptoms I was experiencing. She customised a detox plan that cleared up my digestive problems within a month, and a diet plan that rooted out my recurring infection in a matter of three weeks. What really surprised me was her advice to remove my metal tooth fillings, which proved to be a transformation point not only for my digestive system, but also in terms of my energy levels. I now have much better quality of rest, and am in the second phase of our plan to continue building up the strength of my digestive system. As Sheeba is trained in a variety of therapy techniques, I also benefitted from a cranio-sacral therapy session with her to release tension in my spine. Working with Sheeba has helped me to address my health issues in a comprehensive manner, which I believe will have sustained, long-term benefits. Thank you, Sheeba!

R.P, 29, Private Tutor

CHAPTER 10

INVESTIGATIVE ASSESSMENTS

To discover the internal biochemistry at any point in time, it just makes sense to do the investigative work. But what work would suit your needs? There are many who have already gotten their medical barrage of tests done, done their rounds of hospital corridors and consults, been there and done that...but either have lacked results or frustratingly hit a brick wall.

To illustrate the point here: I met a client who had just started getting migraine attacks that were debilitating. After doing rounds with doctors and MRI scans and more, she was recommended to a specialist doctor, who only saw migraine cases. He gave her some pain medications and upon her asking for an answer as to why she had developed these migraines, he told her that they were "nothing uncommon" and people had worse cases than hers.

Obviously this did nothing to comfort her. The doctor had seen so many cases that he was no longer sensitive to her situation or her fears and concerns. Neither did he answer her question. That's why the word "idiopathic" came into existence—a medical-sounding term meaning, "I don't know how it came to be."

I worked with this client on detoxification, balancing hormones, and eliminating food intolerances. She got completely well, but had to spend her own money, as none of it was covered by her insurance plan. Not everyone can afford to get well in this way, and resort to the dead-end world of (insurance-covered) medications and pills.

For most, including children, it is important to understand, instead, each person's individual biochemistry.

HTMA: Hair Tissue Mineral Analysis: This is a very easy, non-invasive testing method that involves the snipping of some hair close to the roots and sending it off to the lab for analysis. The information it reveals is different from that of a blood test, which tells us what is circulating extra-cellularly (out of the cells) or a urine test that tells us what minerals have been excreted. Only the hair tissue reveals what nutrients the cells absorbed. It even gives indication of the presence of heavy metals.

Functional Blood Assessment: This test can be done by a trained health care practitioner who is able to functionally assess blood test results. They must then identify and assess patterns from the point of view of optimization. This means they are not necessarily trying to diagnose a disease with high and low (red) numbers, but reading between the lines to identify patterns and identify nutrient gaps from the point of view of what's optimal. Basing recommendations with the right diet and supplement protocol is the most fundamental way to start a wellness program, as it helps identify nutrient gaps, excesses, and customizes a complete protocol for the client.

Advanced Blood Chemistry Analysis: This goes beyond just a functional blood test analysis where the summary of the test results very accurately indicates organs or body systems that are stressed. Practitioners can learn how to use this assessment by attending Dr. Kimberly Ballas's (U.S. based) seminars. Just to give some insight into this assessment: I used this for a female client, and it revealed a stressed liver and ovaries. She had not mentioned any hormonal issues to me, so upon questioning her, she was surprised that a blood test picked up this detail. She explained that a long time ago she had polycystic ovaries but had taken some medications and was told that her cysts were now so small that they were not a medical issue. She had forgotten to mention it, as she thought it was a thing of the past. Well, she still needed to work on it, as it was still "there" and manifesting as painful PMS.

Urine Saliva Test: There are several urine saliva tests that measure different things. Some urine tests measure for drugs, infections, heavy metals, pH, or other kidney stress factors. Another urine saliva test (combination) tests for oxidative stress, mineral levels, digestion, detoxification, possible infections, and body pH. Depending on what kind of investigative work needs to be done, these are non-invasive and most times results are immediate. This test would even work for kids.

Hormone Saliva Test: A saliva test is the gold standard in correctly assessing your hormones, whether for cortisol, DHEA, progesterone, or testosterone. Please ask your doctor for this simple non-invasive test rather than the old-fashioned blood test. The free hormones in the saliva give a better indication of real levels in the body rather than the controlled levels in the blood.

Food Allergy Test (Alcat, York, Immupro): Food intolerances are different from food allergies, which you would know right away from the immediate reaction like swelling or rash. Intolerances are a lot more insidious as it's not an immediate reaction to food you have eaten, but a slow one that creates inflammation and digestive unease. I normally do not recommend food allergy tests as they are expensive and not my first choice in terms of protocol; however, it should be done if there are still some unanswered reactions in the body like urticarial (hives). If a person has undergone some detox diet and supporting supplements and has done some heavy metal cleansing and still does not see full results, then it may make sense to carry out this test. I have found that most adults who get the test results have a hard time later following the "avoid" foods as they may be numerous or just not practical. So a person who does the test needs to be ready to alter their eating habits anywhere from two months to sometimes even a whole year.

Bio resonance Scan: This is an energetic and vibrational analysis of all your systems. It is a fairly old test that was developed in Germany to non-invasively carry out a complete bio assessment. This simple device can actually gauge all possible internal physical issues that may exist, energetic and non-harmonious regions that may be causing stress right down to the cellular level. A bio resonance scanner can also "treat" the person by emitting the frequencies that are required to balance these disharmonies. This is a little controversial, but I would recommend it as more of an investigative tool rather than for treatment, based on personal experience.

Zyto Advanced Scan: This is a non-invasive, investigative assessment that produces an immediate report. By measuring the skin's micro current in response to computer stimuli, it helps determine which meridian systems are off, and what is required nutritionally in terms of specific supplements at that point in time. It identifies if you have heavy metals, specific viruses, bacteria and fungus, and many more details that are impossible to gain from regular medical tests. This response changes as the client starts to improve and feel better. The test picks up small changes in the body and is a more effective tool when you are checking for improvement within a month's time for a follow-up session with a client.

I personally use this for kids and adults, as one can't do a blood test every month to assess finer changes in the body. What is most useful is that the Zyto reports are accurate, comprehensive, and self-explanatory to patients. This is not the same as the Compass, which many people use for supplement sales. The advanced software scan is only sold to health-care practitioners.

Genetic Marker Tests: There are a few non-invasive, saliva-based genetic tests available. I find that all genetic tests will be predictable only up to a certain degree. Once you understand that we all have cancer genes, and yes, you may be more prone to a specific cancer because of a strong gene from the family line, you must also know that all genes can be switched ON or OFF–depending on your environment, exposure, attitude, etc. (your epigenetics). The test however, can be more useful in cluing you in on how you should eat and how well your body would respond to specific supplements.

TCM and Ayurvedic Pulse Assessments: The ancient systems of medicine are non-invasive and gentle enough to gauge what systems and meridian pathways are stressed in the body. Based on the person's pulse, enough is revealed to the practitioners to be able to design customized herbs and maybe even a massage, detoxification, or acupuncture protocol. I have found these assessments to be spot on, but whether the protocol plan suits your lifestyle or needs is a different matter. Consistency is key in this form of therapy.

Medical Intuitive: This is a person who can read another person's energy to identify health concerns and issues related to those challenges. One of the most famous medical intuitives is Carolyn Myss, an author of numerous books. My favorite one is *The Anatomy of the Spirit.* So it's not just hocus-pocus, and it saves a person a lot of time and money on hospitals, tests, and doctors.

I personally work with a medical intuitive for my whole family. Sometimes you can't direct your parents to get checked, or get a one year old to do a blood test! So this is an easy way for those who are open to looking at it. Most times it comes up so accurate it can shock you! Medical intuitives are not healers, nor do they claim to be.

Just be cautious and don't believe people who say they can heal you. Only you can choose to heal yourself.

Cancer Test: Try to avoid X-rays, mammograms, MRIs, and other diagnostic scans unless absolutely necessary. They cause a lot of radiation that can create ill health or worsen health. I know it is controversial, as the medical community wants you to do a mammogram every year as a screening. The ugly truth is that the National Cancer Institute reported that among women under 35, Mammography could *cause* 75 cases of breast cancer for every 15 it identifies! The NCI still recommends it and says the benefit outweighs the risks. This would be true if you didn't have any other way of assessing-but that's not the case.

Thermography is a non-invasive, less painful, and radiation free way of getting checked. It also has less false positive readings than mammograms. So why aren't they telling you this? That's for you to think about.

There are very few tests that can accurately identify cancer cells in the body, especially in the early stages. AMAS, or Anti-Malignant Antibody in Serum, can detect cancer cells anywhere in the body with 95 percent accuracy! Most insurance companies can reimburse you for this test. To find a lab, go to www.oncolabinc.com. The test kit is free; the analysis by the lab is about $165.

So why don't people know this? Because it is not yet adopted by mainstream medicine. It was created and researched by a Harvard-trained neurochemist, Dr. Samuel Bogoch, who found a simple solution to identifying common and uncommon cancer molecules.

When I went to see Sheeba, I was desperate for answers and solutions to my health problems. My body had been feeling off for months. My mood was low. I felt exhausted all the time. And then, my hair got really thin and started falling out a LOT more than usual. I knew something was wrong with me, but I didn't know what. I have Hashimoto's thyroiditis and have been told my immune system is low because I get recurring skin infections and upper respiratory tract infections. I have also been battling constipation for the last 20 years.

I sought Sheeba's expertise when my doctor told me my blood test came back "normal". I knew there was something wrong with me and I wanted to find out what it was and treat the cause of it ASAP in an all-natural, holistic manner. Sheeba's blood test analysis opened my eyes to the long list of ailments my body was fighting. From heavy metal toxicity to severe cellular dehydration to borderline anemia to only name a few, no wonder my body was all out of sorts. Needless to say, I started Sheeba's program straight away and have been on the fast road to healing ever since. In less than 2 months, I feel and look much better. I have a more positive and optimistic outlook on life, with higher energy levels, and thicker, healthier hair. I still face constipation issues (a 20yr old problem will rarely disappear right away), but they are slowly getting better and I am looking forward to having regular, healthy bowel movements with no supplemental assistance in the future. I am also aware of what supplements my body now needs for continued healing and maintenance. Thank you Sheeba for helping me turn my health around!

R.P, 37 Yrs, Homemaker

CHAPTER 11

CALCIFICATION

This topic warrants a separate chapter, as understanding this phenomenon can help unravel some health mysteries. It is worth understanding as it relates to heavy metal toxicities and detoxification. It will make you understand why an essential mineral like calcium should not be consumed so readily. I am well aware this is exactly what your doctors and nutritionists tell you to have to prevent bone loss in your senior years.

In the book *The Calcium Lie,* Dr. Robert Thompson explains why it is a myth that we need to increase our consumption of calcium supplements and dairy products.

Our healthy body has a pH of 7.3 (this is the blood we are talking about). When there is an introduction of any toxin into the system via food intolerances, chemical, or heavy metal exposure, the pH alters to being more acidic. This is like an alarm in the body for it to immediately get to work to "douse the fire".

Simple chemistry gets to work with acid plus alkaline substance equaling neutralization. So the body uses the most abundant alkaline mineral it has: calcium, which is stored in the bones. The body will compromise the status of the bones to work on the immediate situation on hand. This calcium helps to neutralize the acid as much as required. Now the body is able to recycle this calcium back to the bones, but it needs a driver to take it there. This "driver" is your vitamin D.

After hundreds of blood tests in tropical Singapore, I have found 100 percent of people low on this nutrient. So, it's very important to take vitamin D if you want to improve calcium levels in your bones.

Another critical point here is that the more toxins you have or are exposed to, the more acidic your pH, which increases calcium loss. Calcium is a mineral in the bone, along with 12 other minerals for bone growth, and its main role is to harden bone tissue. Now if you have excess calcium lying around with no driver to recycle it, then what happens? It starts hardening soft tissue!

What does this mean? Kidney stones, gallbladder stones, bone spurs, arthritic joints, cataracts, arteriosclerosis (hardening of arteries), and the list goes on. Do you get the picture? And if you introduce more insoluble (non-bioavailable) calcium via a supplement into your system, what happens? The situation only gets worse.

So bottom line, even for those with osteoporosis, is to get rid of the toxins causing the acidic pH in the first place. This could be done by clearing up your heavy metals, removing food allergens from your diet, improving circulation through exercise and other therapies, and of course going on a customized detoxification protocol that's right for you. Those on hormone therapy for conditions like thyroid disorders all have osteopenia for the same reasons. Their low progesterone normally sets them up for increased bone loss. It is important to address this with bio-identical hormones. Go to a doctor who you know works with bio-identical and non-synthetic hormones.

For those who genuinely have low calcium, please note that you need 12 other minerals (magnesium, boron, strontium etc.), along with calcium and, of course, good amounts of vitamin D (a normal dose for an adult would be 5,000 IU per day) to actually improve bone and calcium levels.

Once you understand this principle of calcium loss, you will understand why it is so important to maintain an alkaline pH in the body—which you can achieve with the right water, foods, and supplements, as well as detoxification.

Exactly who is susceptible to calcification?

» Those with high stress levels

» Those with amalgam fillings

» Smokers and ex-smokers

» Those taking regular antacids/aspirins

» Those who follow a poor diet consisting of few vegetables and fresh fruits

» Those on multiple medications/drugs

» Those taking soda/soft drinks on a regular basis

NATURAL WAY TO IMPROVE BONE DENSITY:

Look for recipes online for making bone broth. This is made in many traditional cultures where no part of the hunted carcass is left to go to waste. After consuming the flesh, the bones are boiled with vinegar to make a bone broth that is rich in the bone minerals and gelatin. This looks like a thick soup jelly and can be consumed in food or as a soup. It is nutrient dense and is normally made in cultures that do not consume milk; they get all their calcium and nutrient needs from this one source.

Unfortunately, this may not be a choice for vegetarians. Another way, which is a longer process, is to consistently choose alkaline foods in your diet. This prevents the lowering of blood pH that reduces the need for calcium withdrawal from the bones to buffer the pH. That's one of the reasons vegetables and fruits are high on the health list.

Talking about the right supplements, there is only one company I know that has created a bioavailable, plant-based source of calcium and other minerals that corrects calcium and bone deficiencies and addresses issues of hypertension, arthritis, osteoporosis, and the like. More on this will be in the supplement chapter.

I met Ms Sheeba after years of trying to gain weight without any positive results. Just after a 2-week detox and 2 consultation sessions, I managed to have a very healthy diet plan, which not only helps me to gain weight gradually in a healthy way, but also makes me feel more energetic every single day. After consulting with Ms Sheeba, I gained about 3 kg in just one month and my immunity improved a lot. "

David Hoan Dinh, student

CHAPTER 12

CLEANSING

For those dealing with a leaky gut and candida (they go hand in hand), the approach to healing the gut is similar. Even those with skin issues can follow this pattern or approach it initially, as it will benefit almost everyone, including those wanting to lose or gain weight. For cleansing heavy metals, see Chapter 11.

Cleanse: This needs to be done with a candida diet and the right supplements. I would recommend the most restrictive candida diet that should be done over a period of three weeks or more to clear the system. Please note that diet alone does not work; you need to incorporate supplements as well, to support the detoxification systems. I have had people insist on not giving supplements to their children or not taking it themselves (out of fear) and then feeling worse for most of the three weeks. If you are planning to follow the diet, please do support your detoxification pathways. The body is releasing more toxins than normal, and it is really common sense to support this process and not make the body one big garbage dump. Also, please do not think that it means the diet is dangerous to do—it's not, but half-knowledge certainly is.

The Diet: This consists of avoiding, for a period of three weeks or more:

All gluten including bread, wheat, kamut, spelt, oats, rye, barley, all sugar, and variations of sugar, like honey, maple syrup, artificial sweeteners, all fruits, fruit juices, dairy products (milk, cheese, yogurt), potatoes, mushrooms, tomatoes, and corn, all yeast and yeast extract in processed foods, no sauces (including soy sauce), fermented foods like kimchi, miso, etc., no sprouts and sprouted foods, preserved meats, all nuts, seeds, caffeine, and alcohol.

What can be consumed during the diet are foods like rice, millets, quinoa, amaranth, tofu, all other vegetables, coconut (milk, oil, cream, water), avocadoes, all legumes and lentils. I find that butter and ghee seem to be OK for most people despite it being dairy. All other meat, fish, and eggs are fine. All manner of spices, herbs, and greens work well with the program as well. Brown rice pasta, millet pasta or noodles, Bragg's liquid aminos, mustard, and mayonnaise can all be included.

There are no restrictions on how much to eat. Even a child can be put on this diet if need be. The most sensible way to eat is five meals a day, comprised of a hearty breakfast, mid-morning snack, lunch, a mid-afternoon snack, and an early dinner (by 7.30 p.m. the latest). This will help manage blood-sugar levels evenly through the day, creating no highs and lows that tend to manifest as irritability, hunger pangs, cravings, headaches, and more severe forms of hypoglycemia. Please note that after the initial few days, there is a die-off reaction of the fungus, so most people don't feel too well, experiencing general lethargy and a sense of tiredness.

Please also note that all meals and snacks need to incorporate good sources of protein. Refer to the food chapter for more details there.

The reason we need to eat early dinner is so that the body can digest and metabolism is steady. If we don't, the signal to the body is that the calories are not being utilized, and metabolism plummets during sleep, which makes the body think the calories need to be stored (as fat).

I had a client who lost five kilos in a month just by changing this one habit. If a person is staying up late, then a small sensible supper can be consumed at least two hours before bedtime.

What also needs to be mentioned here is that sleeping late or at odd times in the night disrupts the natural detoxification and biorhythm patterns in the body. Normally our detoxification clock starts at 10 p.m. and continues until four in the morning. We really need to follow what we normally instruct our kids to do.

Supplements: There are some general supplements that can be taken with the diet, but customization is best, using a baseline assessment like a blood test.

Probiotic: There are many probiotics in the market, with only five percent of those being effective. That is the ugly truth about supplements in general. I prefer Dr. Xeniji, Dr. Osumex, or Dr. Ohhira brand probiotics, even for toddlers. They are all food-based probiotics that go beyond just being a probiotic culture. They have the prebiotics, the enzymes, and other complex polysaccharides that help the probiotics to stick to the gut. Most people buy probiotics based on the bacteria count in the supplement, e.g., 8,000,000,000 bacteria and so on. The good ones don't need quantity, as quality is enough.

Probiotics are important to improve the gut flora and fauna. Did you know that four pounds of our adult weight is made up of these very bacteria! Also, when we are clearing out overgrowth of bad bacteria and yeast, the space created from this needs to be repopulated with the friendly bacteria that will inhibit the growth of bad bacteria. Friendly gut bacteria also have other functions, like aiding in digestion, absorption, and synthesis of key vitamins and omega fatty acids.

For those who have immune challenges like autoimmune conditions, HIV, cancer, Ebola, MERS (Middle East Respiratory Syndrome) SARS, fibromyalgia, exposure to radiation, chemotherapy, or even those in relatively good health with chronic constipation, you can use a super probiotic called Microbiomax, manufactured in Switzerland. This contains over 42 human strains of bacteria that have over 100 clinically researched scientific papers on their effectiveness. It works beyond a probiotic, as it contains colostrum, which the bacteria help produce more of. So your body produces more of these handy immune cells that can fight all degenerative diseases.

I have personally used this for my family as well as clients with autistic children and immune challenged adults—they found this to be the most effective food-based supplement where there are palpable results. Feedback is that it works better than an antibiotic while making the digestive system feel good!

Digestive Enzymes: Most people would benefit from improved digestion. If you have low stomach acid, apple cider vinegar before each meal can assist to improve stomach pH, or else a full-spectrum digestive enzyme blend will work to completely break down carbohydrates, proteins, fats, and fiber.

Vitamin D3: After testing hundreds of clients for Vitamin D3 in tropical countries like Singapore, I find that everyone is low to very low in their vitamin D status. Most adults need to start taking 5,000 IU every day. It is also the sunshine vitamin. This vitamin is really more a hormone that works to improve calcium levels in bones, and improves immunity and mood.

Iodine: This is the most important mineral, and it can be taken daily in the form of a tablet or a liquid. The amount needed depends on your weight. The average adult can take up to 12.5 mg of iodine. Out of over 80 different trace minerals in the body, this is the only one we need to balance hormones. It also helps to boost immunity, works as a strong antioxidant, as well as for brain health, and to improve detoxification.

Trace Minerals: These are exactly what the name implies: minerals in trace amounts. They are needed in very small amounts in the body for cellular metabolism. I prefer trace minerals that are either plant-derived or from seawater. As much as possible, nature's proportions of minerals are perfect as opposed to taking a man-made trace mineral supplement. The liquids are the best type, as they are most bioavailable. This will immediately work on alkalinizing the body, improving cellular metabolism, and cellular communication. It also supports kidney detoxification.

Liver Detox Phase I and II: Normally, practitioners work on only phase one detox w.r.t. (A part of the liver rather than the entire liver) the liver using milk thistle, B vitamins, and other antioxidants. It is important to support both phases, as in one phase the liver breaks down the toxins, and the other is where the body packages these toxins to be safely excreted by the body. In order to support detoxification of the entire liver, an array of nutrients are required, including all the vitamins, minerals, antioxidants like milk thistle, and green tea in an amino acid base (mostly protein sources from rice or pea that are hypoallergenic for most individuals). This is why this product is available only as a powder rather than a pill. A scoop twice a day is the recommended amount. An example of this would be Mediclear Plus by Thorne Research.

Lymphatic Support: As the liver now has all the nutrients it needs in order to ramp up its entire detoxification pathways, the toxins are packaged and released into the lymphatic system for clearing. It is imperative that there is lymphatic support in order to be able to deal with the overload. I had clients who had gone to other naturopaths who had overlooked this protocol, only to have them getting full on coughs and extremely congested respiratory systems that took a few weeks to clear. Supporting all the detoxification systems is imperative, as the body works together as a symphony, not as a single instrument.

For lymphatic support, a practitioner-grade product is best recommended, as they are strong enough to handle the load. Echinacea Premium from Mediherb or Gtox express from Metagenics work extremely well. Please note that if you do not have access to practitioner-grade lymphatic support, what you buy retail may not be as effective. You would need to increase dosages of retail products to see some effect. Sensibility and caution are what you would need here.

Anti-candida Supplement: An effective anti-candida supplement, preferably practitioner-grade either in the form of homeopathic or herbal, will work well with the program. I have used various types and find that multiple strains of candida in a homeopathic blend work best.

Building: Once you are done with this phase (you can continue this for a few more weeks if you are feeling good), then it is time to move on to the Building phase. This would mean that we include some supplements that can help to soothe and repair the gut lining.

If you know that you have hormonal imbalances, it is good to have teas that help to balance hormones, as they are gentle and soothing. It could be raspberry leaf, red clover, dong quai root, or South American foods like Maca, or Amazon herbs.

Gut-lining Support: There are many great supplements that help to soothe and repair gut lining. Make sure it has L-glutamine, deglycerinated licorice, slippery elm, marshmallow, aloe vera, and glucosamine. This can also help children and adults who have sensitive guts or stomachs, including ulcers.

Adrenal Support: I do recommend most adults use some form of adrenal support. When there is everyday stress for over thirty years, most will need this as it increases energy, vitality, sexual libido, balances hormones, improves circulation, sleep, and more. Look for a reliable brand that has Siberian ginseng (eluthero root) or Korean ginseng, cordyceps, royal jelly with bee pollen, or more. For those dealing with adrenal fatigue, you may need more direct aid like an adrenal glandular product for a short while.

Multi-vitamin Mineral Formula: I do ask my clients to take a clinically efficacious multivitamin and mineral formula. In order to decide which is a worthy one, please read the chapter on supplements that explains how to identify a good one. Please note that once again, it is not worth putting it in your mouth if you aren't sure what you are getting. I have clients who buy Centrum from their local supermarket, and it upsets them when I tell them to throw it away, as it is not even worth finishing the bottle. I will explain why in the Supplement chapter.

Omega 3's: There is a bone of contention here as to whether to take plant-based omegas or fish oils. I would definitely recommend that if you eat fish, please choose fatty fish like salmon, mackerel, trout, etc., that are high in these healthy fats. Then you don't really need to fill in this gap with a supplement.

For vegetarians, this can be tricky getting from vegetarian sources alone, but not impossible. You do need a mix of flaxseed, borage seed, hemp, chia seed oils (or keep rotating with different omega-3 oils), but do incorporate algae, as it contains DHA directly. The body has to go through many enzymatic steps to convert flaxseed (we call them parent oils) into the much-needed brain food EPA and DHA. If for whatever reason there is a miss in any of these enzymatic steps, it means you aren't getting optimum levels of these anti-inflammatory EPA and DHA.

I personally lean towards the brand Green Pastures, which is fermented cod liver and butter oil. The bioavailability of all the nutrients in a food-based blend is what makes the difference.

Fasting: Many believe this to be the ultimate in cleansing and detoxification. I do not advise anyone to do a fast if they can first exercise the option of doing a health practitioner–monitored HCG homeopathic program.

Fasting has shown to work as a powerful anti-inflammatory and therefore reduces disease, which is a manifestation of inflammation in the body. But you compromise your hard-earned muscle stores that tend to get depleted in this process, as a fast works on breaking down and utilizing lean muscle as a calorie source, sparing fat stores which are precious fuel in times of "survival mode" or starvation. The irony is that our toxins are sequestered deep into our fat stores, well away from all metabolically active cells. So is this the ultimate way to detox?

No.

Any protocol or therapy that can mobilize fat stores like infrared sauna, the HCG diet, specific massage techniques, and supplements, all work more effectively to clear up toxins and breaking up fat cells. You cannot recommend a fast to someone who is already underweight (many cancer patients become underweight), but you can recommend a far infrared sauna.

Intermittent Fasting: This is another popular approach and seems to work well for those who need to maintain or lose weight. The approach is to eat in an eight or six hour window, or some just eat once in 12 or 24 hours. Some who follow this also recommend you exercise while in the fasting phase. Many clients of mine who have tried this approach (including myself!) find that they end up feeling hypoglycemic, drained to the point of fatigue after an hour of exercise (usually they don't if they eat). I do not recommend this for diabetics either, although it is said to be particularly useful for them as it increases insulin sensitivity for the same reasons that they can have a dramatic sugar drop, leaving them no choice but to have a quick sugar drink to stabilize levels. This form of dieting works for some, but not for all.

I need to apologize to diehard fans of this fasting protocol, but I find that all forms of fasting promote a sense of lack, desperation, and stress in the body, despite the anti-inflammatory and longevity benefits. I am clearly not a personal fan of this method.

Master Cleanse: This method utilizes fresh lemons, maple syrup, and cayenne pepper to make a pleasant-tasting drink. This is what you drink all day long with no food. It is done for a period of 10 days, after which gradually food is added back into the system.

I have, of course, tried this myself in my excitement to see if I could pinpoint any food reactions or allergies, to clear up my sinusitis and stuffy nose (which I had reason to believe were caused by food intolerances) and see how good I felt after the cleanse. I found it easy enough to follow, but I felt no joy during those 10 days. After, I was still stuck with my allergies, my stuffed nose and sinuses, and no more the wiser on what foods triggered it.

Obviously I was doing it to achieve certain results, which did not occur. It was good to experience it, but I did not derive much health or healing benefits from it—at least not what I was looking for. I would still not write this off as a failure, it just depends what you want to achieve as an end result.

Note: it may be wise to note that if your aim is to lose weight by fasting, after you stop the fasting, the weight comes back on with a vengeance.

Gallbladder Cleanse: Who needs to do this? This is a very effective cleanse to undertake when:

- » You are prone to stone formations like kidney or gall stones
- » You find that you're repeatedly bloated no matter what foods you eat
- » You're anemic
- » You have high uric acid or gout.

» You are a smoker.

These are all good reasons to choose the gallbladder cleanse as it is short, and most people feel and see a difference straightaway which makes it worth doing.

You need to make sure you have two days to yourself when embarking on this cleanse. You need to create a recipe with:

½ cup extra virgin olive oil

2 small grapefruits or 1 large OR juice of 3 lemons

4 tablespoons Epsom salts from pharmacy

2–3 cups water

Mix all together to make a liter of the drink. Keep in the fridge

Breakfast: Have a fat-free, no oil, or cheese breakfast. Keep it light with fruits, boiled egg, yogurt, muesli, or such.

Lunch: Have a fat-free light lunch at noon, after which there is no eating.

2 p.m.: Make sure you have removed one cup of the drink from the fridge to make it room temperature. Drink this mixture. You can have water later, but nothing else.

6 p.m.: Drink another cup of the room-temperature mixture.

8 p.m.: Drink the third cup of this mixture.

9:45 p.m.: Drink the remaining cup of this mixture and immediately lie down in bed. Make sure you sleep on your right side where the liver and gall bladder are located. You may change positions once asleep, which is fine, but the initial position should be on the right side.

You may have loose bowels the next day. Please observe your bowels in case you see greenish or brown stones.

Repeat the same process the second day in exactly the same manner. Please make a fresh batch of the drink. The second day you may find yourself making more trips to the bathroom, which is absolutely normal.

In the next few days, keep to light meals and observe how you feel. This cleanse does not need to be repeated if you are following other protocols mentioned in this book and taking basic supplements every day.

Coffee Enemas: This is an age-old practice, where the person uses one tablespoon of organic coffee boiled in one liter of water and cooled to a tepid temperature. Using an enema bag, this coffee goes up the colon and directly hits the liver and gallbladder. It takes about 12 minutes to do, after which the person empties their bowels almost immediately. There are a few key benefits to doing this at least once a week:

» This reduces systemic levels of toxicity by 700 percent. No supplement can actually work this way, as the caffeinated acids in the coffee bypass the digestive system and stimulate the liver to increase the production of glutathione, the mother antioxidant, or "master detoxifier".

» Coffee enemas eliminate parasites and candida. Many people suffer from these issues, which are difficult to treat. The enema works to fully irrigate and flush the liver and colon.

» They detoxify and help to repair the liver. People who have constant bloating and poor digestion can all benefit from this. In fact, it is the number-one recommended therapy for those who have any kind of cancer.

» Coffee enemas cleanse and heal the digestive tract and improve healthy gut peristalsis without disrupting healthy gut flora. Helps to quickly move toxins and debris from liver and out the colon.

» Coffee enemas improve mood and mental clarity. The coffee helps to stimulate bile production and flow, increases oxygen transfer, and stimulates the effective removal of waste. All this makes the body more efficient, uplifting mood to boot.

» Coffee enemas help to relieve chronic pain and ease detox symptoms. This was discovered in World War I, when morphine was in short supply, and the nurses would rely on enemas to ease soldiers' pain.

» Coffee enemas are an inexpensive and effective way to move toxins out of the body quickly. It is a quick healer and prevents the body from having chronic illness.

Saltwater Flush: This is a relatively simple flush that many can do without feeling queasy. It works better than a colonic irrigation, and it works on the entire gut, not just the colon. It can be done a few times a week if required, and is especially good for those who have chronic constipation. This method can be done for just one day or several days in a row, and it helps to clear out the digestive tract in one swoop.

You need to take one tablespoon of either Celtic sea salt or pink Himalayan salt and mix it in one liter of water. Add a squeeze of lemon (depends on taste) and then first thing in the morning, upon waking, gradually drink the entire liter. Go at your own doable pace. You do not eat anything. Once you have finished the one liter, you will find that you need to go to the toilet several times, with the last few having only water coming out. You will find a period where there will be no more bowel movements. It is imperative that you drink and hydrate yourself with more water throughout the day as this flush leaves one very dehydrated, as you have lost a lot of internal water as well.

You can eat your meals as per normal after that.

Who needs to do it? When you don't want to do any sort of colonic irrigation, but want to do a simple home cleanse to clear your colon.

It works for those who get constipated once in a while or who have come back from a trip/holiday and want to clean up. Helps with bloating, gas, and acts as a cleanse after unhealthy eating.

It can be done for a few days in a row if required.

Castor Oil Pack: This is not really a cleanse, but does fall under the detoxification category. It is a simple, inexpensive, yet powerful tool to use. It works to pull out toxins from a localized area while improving circulation and stimulating the lymphatic system to clear out toxic waste. It can be done as often as one desires, as there are no side effects, and it is done externally, so it does not interfere with any possible medications either.

You need to have cold-pressed castor oil, which you can use to soak a cotton or flannel cloth (the size depends on the area you want to cover). Place this oiled cloth on a sheet of plastic. Place the oiled cloth on the area, e.g., abdomen, and then lay the plastic over it. Over the plastic, you need to place a hot water bottle for a hot compress effect. Keep this for an hour and remove. This can be repeated daily or as often as is necessary.

Who needs it?

» Those who have some insect bite or unknown swelling

» Women with fibroids, cysts, or endometriosis

» Eye swelling, bug bites, bee stings

» Skin irritations

It removes toxins effectively and without feeling any side effects. It stimulates lymph to clear out the toxins.

Enzyme Drinks: Now there are many fermented vegetable and fruit drinks available in the markets, which have multiple benefits. The good ones contain high antioxidants, plant collagen, active cultures, and enzymes that help the body cleanse and detox at the cell level. These drinks are food-based cultures so all ages can have them. Depending on how much you take, it can have a bowel-cleansing effect or cellular detox effect, as some may be energizing, while others are nourishing. I prefer such cultures to someone resorting to laxatives. The good ones come from the MLM companies or network marketing companies, who are confident of their product as many are mentioned in the *Physician's Desk Reference*. These fermented drinks are more in the Asian cultures, like Japan and Taiwan, so I prefer companies from these locations, like Avita, which has its manufacturing plant in Taiwan. What you need to research is how many days it has been fermented for, what vegetables/fruits have been used, and maybe even herbs that are blended to produce a powerful product. Such products can enhance metabolism, detoxify, enhance skin and complexion, nourish with antioxidants, and provide *prebiotic* (foods that support probiotic growth) rich culture.

I like these drinks, as they are not hard-core like a colonic, and can even be given to children with digestive unease or to clear their bowels. They taste very good and the dose can be adjusted to suit individual needs. Some brand names are Nutrabiotics and Vita 18.

Having battled with infertility for many years and having gone through countless fertilit treatments, I came to Sheeba at my heaviest in May 2014. Sheeba did an extensive analysis of my state of health and suggested many "doable" lifestyle changes with the weight loss program. All supplements I was recommended were natural and I did not get any side effects which was amazing considering how sensitive and toxic a system I had. In 3 months I lost 12 kilos and kept it off. My complexion and energy levels were amazing. My monthly periods returned 1 month into the diet and my cycle was back to normal after 5 years of being unpredictable. In September this year, we found out I was 4 weeks pregnant!! Naturally without fertility drugs! Sheeba helped me achieve something so close to my heart and I'm forever thankful! Thank you Sheeba!

R. C, Human Resources, 32 yrs

CHAPTER 13

HEAVY METAL CHELATION

nflammation, pain, candida, allergies, skin conditions, all hormonal imbalances, autism, and autoimmune diseases are all linked to heavy metal poisoning.

Clinical trials and scientific referenced articles have found that, among many other things:

» Heavy metal chelators work to break up the bio film of yeast and fungus, including candida. This means it is a more powerful antifungal than antifungal medications.

» They work similar to, or are more powerful than antibiotics, and can disrupt antibiotic-resistant bacteria growth, and aid in quick recovery from infection(s).

» They work like strong free-radical quenchers and anti-inflammatories, thus reducing chronic pain and disease issues. Remember, inflammation is the basis for any disease.

» They retard muscle cramping and pain, as heavy metals are a large source of this in the first place.

» They clear up and prevent further calcification, thus helping to clear up calcium stones and calcified arteries, and promoting circulation and heart health.

» Usage of heavy metal chelators has improved cancer recovery and outcomes by 90 percent.

» Improves diabetes and blood sugar imbalances, including insulin resistance.

» Improves the endocrine system or all hormonal responses in the body, reducing hormone therapy.

» Improves mood, mental clarity, and memory.

As you can see, a heavy metal chelation would benefit anybody! We are all exposed to it, so even regular healthy people can benefit from a detox like this.

You can start with any water filter system that can clean up heavy metal and organic chemicals in water. You also seriously need to consider a shower filter, as you do absorb chlorine and metals from your bath, transdermally.

A very simple and inexpensive way to get rid of heavy metals is by using a far infrared sauna or a far infrared sauna blanket that can be used at home.

Supplements can work well with this program to create a faster and more effective cleanse.

There are very few oral heavy metal chelators in the market. Other oral metal detoxes work superficially. The body needs to be detoxed in layers, so it needs to be done over at least a three-month period or more, depending on the severity of the situation.

Biotics Research is a company that has an oral supplement called **Porphyra-zyme** or now renamed Chela-zyme.

Another effective oral detoxifier is Stem Detox. You normally don't need to know what exact heavy metal toxicities you have, as they are normally hidden away in layers. These heavy metal detoxifiers would work on the initial layers. Deeper layers sequestered into brain tissue, fat stores, bones, and organs take longer and deeper work.

Specifically for those dealing with mercury toxicity, no one knows their research and work quite like Dr. Chris Shade, a global expert on mercury toxicity and clearing. The supplements specifically work by getting all the mercury out of your system.

An expensive proposition is to get a heavy metal chelation using IV—which means getting it done through an integrated doctor who can set you up on a drip for an hour or more. Ozone therapy seems to work in a similar manner, and will bind to all free radicals including heavy metals. It also works to purify blood, and get the much-needed oxygen into your cells, which heavy metals all the while have deprived.

Another option that bypasses the digestive system like the IV, is to use an anal suppository. The good ones make sure that they have glutathione in there, along with EDTA (heavy metal chelators), to quench all free radicals and prevent your liver enzyme numbers from spiking due to the removal of heavy metals from the body. This also prevents a detoxing effect that can leave you sapped when heavy metals are passing out of the body. It is good to take with activated charcoal to prevent recirculating the toxins into your digestive tract. **Tox detox** or **Detoxamin** are clinically proven to work in this regard. For those who need a gentler approach (for example, anyone who has active cancer), use **Modifilan,** a brown seaweed that helps reduce side effects of chemotherapy and radiation (even from Chernobyl radiation—they gave this to those exposed to the reactor with great results), which also helps in self-destruction of the cancer cells to boot.

I would like to mention that parents who are looking at products that will work for children need to see which one suits the child, depending on age, swallowing capabilities, and what's practical, as the liquid oral ones smell and taste quite bad and are difficult to mask in drinks. There are some homeopathic heavy metal detox complexes that aid in cleansing, like **CH77** and **IMD powder** from **Quicksilver**, for specific mercury detox. Normally these are practitioner products, recommended by health care practitioners familiar with heavy metal chelation. If you have just had your amalgam fillings replaced, you do need to go through the leaky gut protocol, along with taking IMD powder and glutamine powder. Please see respective chapters 7 & 8 on this.

It would be sensible to support your system with a good lymphatic cleanser like Gtox Express, a multi-vitamin and chelated mineral complex, including antioxidants like liposomal vitamin C, liposomal B vitamins, magnesium, and trace minerals.

During this phase of heavy-metal cleansing, it is essential to support the adrenal system, that can get stressed and fatigued due to movement of these heavy metals. Take some herbs like ginseng, cordyceps, Siberian ginseng, royal jelly, and super foods like spirulina, and cracked wall chlorella, which work well during a heavy metal detox. They help to clear out the heavy metals quicker from the body so it has a less negative impact.

I will talk about supplement support in detail in the next chapter.

Since being diagnosed with Hidradenitis Suppurativa 8 years ago, I have seen numerous dcotors, dermatologists, plastic surgeons and even a gynaecologist. Nothing worked for me and my flare ups were worse than ever. I had just about given up and committed myself to living a life of pain and humiliation when I read about Sheeba. She truly was God sent. She recommended something so simple but overlooked by the other doctors I'd seen — a blood test! Through that, she knew exactly what was mising in my body and what was going wrong and prescribed me the right supplements. I also embarked on the Hcg Diet as I was overweight and I lost around 8 kg in 6 weeks! My HS wound in my inner thigh has completely healed and my wounds in the underarms are in the process of complete healing. having suffered 8 years with open wounds and bleeding lesions, I am overwhelmed with how pain- free I am now. Thank you Sheeba for everything and always being professional yet caring and sympathetic- qualities many professional doctors lack. Thank you for also being just a phone call or text away when I needed clarification or advice."

Gayathri N, 27 yrs

CHAPTER 14

THYROID – EVERYONE IS SUSCEPTIBLE

There are many books written on thyroid problems. I am dedicating an entire chapter to it, as this is one of the most common issues I see when working with my clients.

Thyroid experts like Dr. Denis Wilson and Dr. Thierry Hertoghe believe that 80 percent of the adult population has an underactive thyroid and doesn't know it. Most have a subclinical situation, meaning it will not reflect in a blood test. A blood test is not a good measure for any hormones to begin with (please see chapter on Assessments). Many people experience adrenal fatigue that can create an underactive thyroid. What does this really mean? How do I know if I am susceptible?

Here are some signs and symptoms that clue you in:

» If you are a smoker or an ex-smoker

» If you have depression, bipolar disorder, or OCD (obsessive-compulsive disorder)

» Joint stiffness, carpal tunnel syndrome

» Hypertension or low blood pressure

» High cholesterol and high blood lipids

» Diabetes, Parkinson's, Alzheimer's

» Miscarriages and premature birth

» Pregnancy complications and birth defects

» Vertigo or tinnitus

» Sleep apnea, insomnia

» Arthritis and other inflammatory diseases

» Eczema, psoriasis, skin allergies, rashes

» Puffy hands and feet, muscle/joint pain

» Constipation, puffy eyes, or eye bags

» Irregular menses, frequent muscle cramps

» Low sex drive/impotence/infertility/PCOS/fibroids

» Varicose veins, poor circulation

» Rapid heartbeat, palpitations, feeling cold

» Recurring anemia, low iron

» Thinning hair, thinning outer third of eyebrows

» Increased body fat/visceral fat, loss of muscle mass

» Reduced attention span, calculation, memory issues

» Parents with autistic children or with learning disabilities

» Parents whose baby on mother's milk develops eczema

A simple way to find out if you have an underactive thyroid is by doing a basal body temperature test for three or four days. As soon as you wake up, take your temperature under your armpit. If the readings each day are below 98.6 degrees Fahrenheit, this may be all you need to indicate an underactive thyroid.

The most accurate way to test for thyroid issues is a Thyroflex test. This test is a physical one, which takes five minutes, and is completely non-invasive. It tests your reflex and correctly gauges if you have a hyper or hypothyroid situation. This is really for those who need a black and white diagnosis before they will start helping themselves. For others, starting from the beginning by correcting diet, taking customized supplements, heavy metal chelation, and taking adrenal or thyroid support would be essential to getting better. And yes, it is reversible, no matter what the doctors tell you, including autoimmune thyroid conditions.

Please note, that for those already taking thyroid medication, it is a synthetic form of the T4 hormone. When you have an underactive thyroid, what the body needs is to convert this T4 to an active T3. But, unfortunately for some, the body is unable to make this conversion, so the thyroid medication is not very useful. Instead, what you can do is go to a doctor who will prescribe you natural thyroid medications which contain all the thyroid hormone complexes of T1, T2, T3, and T4. This is a more natural and balanced support for those who need hormone support. Some brand names are Armour Thyroid, Nature Thyroid, and more.

Who is more susceptible?

» Smokers and ex-smokers

» Those with adrenal fatigue

» Those exposed to radiation, like disaster zones or pilots/stewards

» Those with amalgam teeth fillings

» Athletes who do intense sports or marathons

» Women during pregnancy or post delivery if proper nutrients are not restored

» Those whose parents have amalgam fillings

» Those who've been exposed to mercury and heavy metals through food/contamination

» Everyone who drinks fluoridated water or showers/swims in chlorine pools regularly

---

Did you know?

That German researchers found that 80% of the adults who developed cancer also had an underactive thyroid. The thyroid gland is essential for metabolism, hormone health, immunity and more.

I came to Sheeba to find a solution for chronic fatigue, after months of tweaking my sleep patterns and diet and taking alternative medicine without success. I was immediately drawn to Sheeba's principles of practice and her friendly disposition. From the results of my comprehensive blood test, Sheeba identified many areas of deficiency and imbalance, and prescribed specific supplements and homeopathic medicine to overcome them. I appreciate her approach of analyzing the blood test results using an optimum health range; a GP had dismissed my case as the blood test results were in the 'correct range' according to allopathic standards, although I was far from feeling vital. Within a few weeks of following Sheeba's recommendations, my energy gradually returned. I am relieved to find a solution and thankful to arrest the deficiencies at an early stage. I look forward to working with Sheeba in years to come, and highly recommend her to anyone seeking vibrant health!.. G H , Editor,

Female, 31yrs

CHAPTER 15

SUPPLEMENTS

Everyone has a unique biochemistry, so what each person needs is different, whether it is from food, diet, or supplement plan. But, like an umbrella insurance plan, there are some things that can be generalized. There are many books available on each of these that we now know to be essential for health. Some worth mentioning are: *The Calcium Lie, The Sunshine Vitamin, The Miracle Mineral: Magnesium, Iodine: Why We Need It and Why We Can't Live Without It, Trace Minerals, Water and Salt.*

Let me also clarify here that RDA amounts of vitamins are archaic and valid only enough to prevent disease and are not formulated for *optimal health,* nor is RDA based on age requirements. That is why nutritionists like to call it the Ridiculous Dietary Allowance, because it is really a joke.

All supplements are not created equal. Unfortunately, 90 percent of what's available on the shelves and market today just won't cut it— or worse, may be crap. Most supplements are not bioavailable, which means that the body is unable to absorb them. The best types are the ones that are more bioavailable. Now that we know that, what bioavailable supplements are actually worth taking?

Before I answer this, a question I get a lot is: Do we need to take supplements for life? The answer to that is a resounding yes. It's only when you are not in an urban environment or exposed to everyday toxicities that you don't need any additional support.

I also get this a lot: "Oh, my grandfather never took any pills, and he lived to be 100!" Yes, he did. He also probably ate mostly home food, didn't travel much, and wasn't exposed to the multitude of toxins and radiation from technology, and the added stress to boot.

Another favorite is "When should kids start taking supplements?" This is a tricky one, as it is very important to always inculcate good food habits and to make sure you are exemplifying healthy eating habits, as they emulate their elders and what they see in their family setting. If your kids fall sick often due to school exposure, then starting early to boost the immune system is a good idea. But giving them supplements that are in the form of gummies or sweet liquids is not the right way to do it.

Children: For children, I would start with getting them involved in the kitchen. Begin with getting them to make some pure fruit puree ice-lollies. Educate them as to why these are better than a regular ice cream. Progress to getting them to create some smoothies with fresh fruit, and add some super food powder mix. Get real foods like cacao powder, not the supermarket chocolate powder. These are all super foods that taste delicious and kids want more of. When they make it themselves, they are interested in trying it.

Get them used to swallowing pills rather than buying the chewy supplements, which are normally avoidable, due to their sugar content and poor efficacy value. Most of the time, pills you need to swallow don't have sugar. Some liquid multi-vitamins and mineral food-based supplements are very good; they need to be refrigerated after opening and have a short shelf life. I prefer Floradix brand, but now there are many other good ones on the market without the added sweeteners and preservatives. This liquid supplement can be used for children up to four years old, after which you need to try and switch them to swallowing capsule-type supplements or powders that make a decent tasting drink.

I have many clients who believe in "going natural" and putting natural things into their body rather than taking any kind of pill—whether it's a medication, supplement, food-based product, or herb.

Considering all the exposure to toxicities and processed foods, we really are not living "naturally." Tribal people are the closest to this description, and their communities have been studied for their robust health and intuitive knowledge.

In an urban setting, knowledge on the correct kind of supplements can work as a health insurance plan. It may be an expensive choice to make, but once you are sick, not only are the expenses overwhelming, but also for many, you pay for the rest of your life.

Preventive care is the best gift you can give yourself and your family.

There are many supplements out in the market. How do you know which one is for you? If you can get professional-grade supplements from your nutritionist or naturopath, that is going to be of better value for your money, as practitioner-grade costs the same as regular supplements, but are generally better formulated for best absorption. Another option is network companies that sell supplements, because their products are better quality than most retail. Do your research, as some companies use anecdotal references, while others have actual clinical studies done, and their supplements are mentioned in the PDR or *Physician's Desk Reference*.

Here I would like to mention my inspiration, Dr. Joel Wallach. He was a veterinary doctor (now a naturopathic doctor), who studied animals of all types, including humans—he performed hundreds of autopsies and did decades of research. He has won several awards and medals for his research and work in this field. What he found was that *all* diseased states stem from some nutritional deficiency or other—animals and humans alike. He has challenged the medical community with this, and has proven many times over, that with the right supplements and diet, disease is reversible and can be eradicated. He also believes that exercising without supplementation is equivalent to suicide! I highly recommend his book: *Dead Doctors Don't Lie.*

Wallach has created state-of-the-art supplements—the best on the planet in my opinion, for all age groups as well as those with compromised health, digestion, and sensitivities.

His supplement line is called Youngevity, and works on the networking model. This is my first choice of supplements for anyone, where results are inevitable, due to their high quality and bioavailability.

Most supplements are not so well absorbed in the body—even foods we eat are digestion compromised. A good supplement will be absorbed by 20 to 25 percent if you are lucky. Liquids work better for this reason, as well as food-based supplements. Sublingual supplements have a distinct advantage, as they bypass the digestive tract entirely. There are some suppository-based supplements available that do exactly that, but most healthy people prefer not to use that route. Normally, only those with severely compromised digestion use suppository-based supplements.

Another way to get specific nutrients is via IV, but again, that is for those looking at high doses or need immediate attention.

So it boils down to a lot of swallowing at the end of the day. What do you need to look out for in a supplement?

» **Organic Compounds:** Make sure all ingredients are completely listed. For example, Centrum multivitamin mentions a list of minerals, e.g., Calcium, but does not state what calcium compound it is. They should clearly specify: calcium carbonate. If this most basic information is missing, you have no idea what you are getting, what you are ingesting, and what the quality or bioavailability of the product is. I would steer clear, as the manufacturer is hiding basic information, which may induce more toxicity in the body if consumed.

» **Too many ingredients:** You feel good when you see a supplement that lists multiple ingredients, thinking you will get so much more out of the product than a regular one. An example of this is a Men's Multi formula, which has other herbs and antioxidants in it, along with the generic multivitamin, and mineral blend. Beware of this, as there are so many ingredients, that you get a little of everything that really amounts to nothing. Always go for a generic multivitamin mineral formula, rather than gender specific with additional blends.

» **Multi-vitamins:** For all good multivitamins (not supplements in general, but a good, everyday multi-nutrient formula), there are many companies that entice with "One-a-day" versions. This is a complete myth. If you want to meet RDA levels (Recommended Daily Allowances, aka what nutritionists call Ridiculous Dietary Allowances), then yes, it will suffice. The really good ones will ask you to take a minimum of three tablets a day or more. If this doesn't work for you, there are excellent powdered versions available that are not high on the taste test, but are palatable with some rice/almond milk and a fruit smoothie, or stick to the Youngevity brand for their 90+ nutrient formula.

» **Sugars:** No good supplement will have any fillers or taste enhancers. Read all ingredients on the labels. The more "fillers" or non-active ingredients they have, the more you need to avoid them. Point to note here is to always go for swallowing capsules rather than the chewable types, which have unnecessary ingredients to make it taste good. Powder is even better than capsules.

» **Bioavailability:** The most important aspect of selecting a supplement is to know what forms are bioavailable to the body. Calcium as calcium carbonate is as good as eating chalk. The body does not recognize these inorganic compounds of sulphate, oxide, chloride, carbonate etc.—They are almost useless. What your body recognizes and puts to use are organic compounds, like mineral amino acid chelates, that are teamed with an array of minerals or specific nutrients to work like a "complex", rather than one single nutrient. For example, it has been proven that Vitamin C is better utilized and absorbed by the body when it is combined with citrus bioflavonoids. This is called vitamin C complex. B vitamins, like Cyanocobalamin, are actually toxic. Please choose the Methylcobalamin version instead.

» **Food-based:** Choose real food-based supplements where possible, e.g., instead of choosing a whey protein isolate, choose brown rice 98 percent bioavailable protein powder. This is still a whole food rather than an isolate or single ingredient/extract.

» **Practitioner range:** If you are looking at improving health, then most of these retail supplements are just not strong enough or clinically effective. For years, I was taking echinacea to boost my immunity, but never found it to work. When I was introduced to practitioner-grade Medi-Herb Echinacea, I was stunned. In one dose, I felt the difference!

» **Iron:** A word of caution is never to take iron tablets without getting a blood test done to confirm that you are low in iron. It is toxic and harmful to have excess iron in your blood.

» **Calcium:** As mentioned in the Calcification chapter, most people should take only the right type of calcium. When you do, make sure you add at least 5,000 IU of vitamin D to that, and there are many minerals that combine with the calcium in the supplement to give you a "complex".

» **Liposomals:** Vitamin C and other products like glutathione are not well utilized by the body. They have a quick half-life, meaning they are very quickly removed in the urine, and don't stay active for very long. This effect is important if you are ill. Some recommend taking 1,000 mg of Vitamin C by the hour when a person is sick. But the side effect of this is loose bowels, as it is not well tolerated. All of this can be avoided by simply using a liposomal version of the product. It is extremely well tolerated, even at high doses, stays in the body a longer time, and is thus more effective. You automatically need to consume less for this reason. It is a pricier option, but is worth the money. These forms of delivery are far superior to others. Liposomal versions are emulsions that are soluble in water or fats. This works to your advantage, as it stays longer in the body and is thus better utilized, as opposed to ascorbic acid, which very quickly flushes out in the urine. These are more expensive than the traditional vitamin C's, but you need less and the body uses more. It's just smart supplementation.

» **Super PEO'S:** These are plant essential oils that are extracted from fruits like berries, flowers, and fruits that have a very high antioxidant value, unlike any other foods. These are wonderful for the elderly, those who have increased antioxidant needs from surgery, chemotherapy, or just from malaise, and recovering from a bad bout of illness. They are under the super-food oil category, and taking a little every day would benefit all.

» **Derma Fusion Technology:** Now there are products using enhanced technology called Derma Fusion, which are skin patches that you stick on. There are specific nutrients in there that have a 24-hour time release. This smart supplementation bypasses the digestive tract, so it's 100 percent bioavailable, compared to a regular pill or powder. The specific brand that sells this is Thrive Premium Lifestyle.

» **Multi-Level Marketing Products:** Generally speaking, I favor these network marketing products, as you are getting better quality than what retail offers in the supplement category. But buyers beware, and make sure you do your homework, to ensure that the supplements are mentioned in the *Physician's Desk Reference*. Most of these companies put more money on the research and quality of the product versus marketing, but because of their networking strategy, they can be pricy.

» **Nanotechnology:** This is taking the world by storm in many industries. There are supplements that use this innovation, so the body doesn't really need to break it down. It is almost immediately available, and improves absorption even in digestion-compromised individuals.

» **Rotation:** Once you feel you have found the right brand, most would stick to it. I recommend that some supplements be changed every now and then like multivitamins, minerals, omega-3 fats, and herbal supplements you may be taking. This is a good time to become aware, in case something was not suiting you. It also helps you to get nutrients from different sources, like omega-3 from plants, fish, or krill. This is the same reason that we need to eat different fruits and vegetables: so we get an array of nutrients from different sources. The same goes for skin care or personal care products. It also helps prevent exposure to the same toxicities/sensitivies from the same products, if any.

WHAT SUPPLEMENTS TO TAKE?

According to Dr. Joel Wallach, we need 90+ nutrients to build a foundation for good health. That would include all the vitamins, over 70 minerals, and 12 amino acids as a start. That is included in his Beyond

Tangy Tangerine powder. The other critical supplement for long term bone health and a body pH balancer is the Osteo Fx powder. This has over 70 plant-derived minerals, along with calcium, and Vitamin D for bone health, repair, and all cell metabolisms.

Your supplement list would look something like this on most days:

Please note that supplements should always be based on the weight of the person, so dosage would vary based on size.

For adults:

Vitamin D: total of up to 5,000 IU/day

Iodine: 600–1,200 mcg/day

Beyond Tangy Tangerine: based on body weight

Osteo Fx: complete calcium (with 72 plant-based minerals) based on body weight

Omega-3 oils: 2-3 caps (up to 3,000 mg/day)

Liposomal Vitamin C: This would vary depending on strength of product and how well you are feeling that day.

Then, depending on your health, you may want to add or layer your supplements, eg., if you have osteoarthritis, you may want to add Glucogel (a Youngevity supplement for improving bone matrix) to the above list, and so on.

If you have pets and are feeding them packaged or canned food, please note that they do need supplements for optimal health. They can benefit with almost the same supplements as humans, except that the dose is based on their body weight. Animal probiotics are available and can be given from time to time as required.

When I first arrived in Sheeba's office I was exhausted and entirely drained from seeing so many different medical practitioners. I was suffering from a chronic fatigue that made everything seem like a chore. In addition to this, I was also dealing with excessive thirst, damaged vocal chords, constant headaches, sore muscles and joints and extremely bad blood work.

As a 25 year old Primary School teacher who hates being sick, I'd spent years convincing myself that it was normal to return home from work too tired and drained to consider doing anything. I was sleeping for as many hours as possible, never felt rested and would frequently cry from sheer exhaustion. As the months passed and I failed to improve I eventually took myself to see the GP. After 27 doctors appointments, numerous tests and scans and a spiraling list of diagnoses, none of which seemed related, I felt overwhelmed by everything I was being told and the fact that no one was able to connect them all together. That was, until, my appointment with Sheeba.

Fast forward a few months and with Sheeba's guidance I now feel better than ever. I have a clarity of thought that I have never experienced before and endless amounts of energy. I wake up in the morning and no longer feel like crying because I'll have to make it through the entire day without going back to bed. Most importantly for me, I have the energy to want to do things. I want to do well at my job, I want to spend time with my friends and visit my family. All those around me have noticed a difference and many have commented on how much better I look, most notably the 'sparkle in my eyes'.

Sheeba has given me a new sense of life and for that I can't thank her enough. At 25 I finally feel like I'm living and I'm so excited about what life will bring.

L.W, Female, 25 yrs.

CHAPTER 16

SUPPORT FOR ALL BODY SYSTEMS

Pituitary: This is the gland that sits right behind your third eye area. Many clients report recurring pain in just that area. This is an indication that the pituitary gland is trying to manage the "situation."

Positive: The pituitary gland is positively sensitive to trace minerals, iodine, potassium, HCG (homeopathy), and essential oils like sandalwood.

Negative: It is sensitive to toxins (heavy metals), any endocrine gland inflammation, hormonal imbalances, and low minerals. Clearing toxins and adding nutrients via food and supplements is the best way to support the pituitary.

Pineal: If assessments reveal that the pineal gland is in overdrive, it indicates the person has high anxiety, depression, or panic attacks.

Positive: It's sensitive to heavy metal detox, chemical/environmental detox, ginseng, Suma herb, and golden seal. Lavender essential oil works well to calm.

Negative: This gland is affected by toxicities and low grade infections/inflammation.

Well supported by craniosacral therapy, meditation, and removal of fluoride exposure.

Hypothalamus: This is another master gland, like the pituitary.

Positive: Affected by potassium, trace minerals, iodine, thyroid hormones/support, super greens like chlorella, and organic sulphur (MSM).

Negative: Affected by poor mineral status, toxicities, and underactive thyroid. An essential oil that stimulates this gland is geranium.

Neurotransmitters: Neurotransmitters are chemical compounds that communicate with the brain. You may have heard of dopamine or serotonin. Yes, if not optimal, it can cause depression and sleep disturbances. So how does one work on neurotransmitters? You definitely need to work on your digestive system if you need to improve these neurotransmitters (please read chapter on the second brain), but there are some specific supplements that may work. I personally like to work with energetic medicine for something so sensitive, and most people are already taking some form of medication, so therapeutic grade essential oils or homeopathic remedies will not interfere with that.

Remedy: Almost all essential oils work on neurotransmitters. Depending on the issue (sleep, depression, anxiety, etc.), you can choose which essential oil will work best. Some immediate choices would be orange, lavender, peppermint, neroli, lemon, etc.

There are several practitioner Desbio products that can help balance neurotransmitters. But there are some supplements like L-tryptophan, SAM (S-adenosylmethionine), and liver cleansers like Mediclear Plus (Thorne Research), that can help to improve—remember, again, it's working on the digestive and clearing out toxicities that make the difference.

Note: Check for an underactive/subclinical thyroid condition if there are neurotransmitter challenges like sleep or depression issues. Liver cleanse is essential.

Head: You will be surprised to know that although we get headaches, there are no pain sensors in the brain! Research has proven that peppermint oil can relieve a headache just as quickly as a paracetamol, without the side effects of taking a medicine. In fact, it works on most types of headaches. Migraines are a little more complex, as there is a correlation with liver toxicity, food sensitivities, and hormones. However, if you have had any head falls or impact at any age (or if you are into boxing), please do choose to go for craniosacral therapy, as it helps to release old compressions that can impact the flow of chi or energy.

Remedy: There are very few drugs and foods that can cross the blood-brain barrier, but as for cellular hydration, essential oils can all work in restoring balance. I would choose frankincense, sandalwood, myrrh, galbanum, and spikenard as some of the essential oils to work with in this area.

Sinus: These are hard-to-reach areas, so it can be tricky to work with clearing them up. Most people suffering from sinus issues will have some food intolerances as well. Most are given multiple doses of antibiotics to clear the infection. The majority of sinusitis issues are not bacterial, but *fungal.* That's why antibiotics generally make it worse, and it comes back with a vengeance.

Remedy: You need to take anti-candida or tailor made homeopathic supplements for sinus-like Sanum Remedies or Desbio, both practitioner homeopathic ranges. You can also use Smart Silver or Argasol silver 30 ppm, and drop a few drops into the nostrils or even put one teaspoon in a neti pot of water and use that to flush out the sinus area. Xlear nasal spray works well for some to clear the sinuses. Due diligence definitely pays off here. A good lymphatic mover would work to help keep the sinus clear of congestion and phlegm buildup. These could be herbs like cleavers, sarsaparilla, echinacea, or a combination of such, in a tea or pill base. Physical lymph drainage using the Nuskin body/face spa is effective to drain sinus and congestion areas.

Eyes: If you have eye itchiness, please use a lymphatic cleanser, as that can immediately clear the congestion/irritants that cause the itchiness, whether it is due to allergy or infection.

Remedy: If you have an eye infection, you can use 10 or 30 ppm (I prefer the higher strength) silver Argasol and just put a couple of drops in each eye twice or thrice a day. It is completely safe and effective. Another simple solution is to use Boric acid powder (available in general stores or health stores), and add ¼ teaspoon to a bowl of distilled water. Use sterile cotton to dip into this solution, and gently apply to closed eyelids. This is a natural anti-bacterial that will help clear infection rapidly and prevent spreading of the infection.

Skin: Everyone's skin is different and hence reacts differently. So what would suit most people across the board? I find that there are a few solutions that can work for even the most sensitive skin, or weepy eruptions.

» First, please use a liver and lymphatic support to detoxify, as these two are directly related to skin. You can use products I have mentioned in earlier chapters.

» If you are working on young ones, please use homeopathic remedies or herbal teas that will work similarly.

» Leaky gut is another culprit, so look into that (please read digestion chapter). For application, you can use Argasol or Smart Silver gel that will help quicken healing, even for third-degree burns.

» You can read the chapter on light spectrochrome for speeding up healing if it is all over the body.

» Another gentle, yet powerful product is medihoney, or raw manuka honey, of at least 15 umf strength. Direct application on open wounds can work wonders.

» High strength Vitamin E (70,000 IU) oil application directly to skin scars is effective in quick healing and clearing up scars

» If you have a serious skin infection, then applying essential oils may be warranted, but please ask for professional advice, as using essential oils the right way is important, else it can make things worse.

» Most aloe vera gels do not contain active ingredients, but if you can use the actual fresh plant, that is best. If you can get the aloe bitters, applying and ingesting that is extremely effective. If not, make sure the product you are using states it has a specific strength of activity.

» Hydration is key for good skin, so make sure you are drinking more than enough water.

Hair: I find hair is a sensitive one for many people—women and men both experience thinning hair. It is not inevitable as men think, based on genes. It can be completely reversed naturally, as long as you have hair cells and are not completely bald.

» You do need to work on yourself internally to clear out toxins, but we need to work on improving direct circulation to the head, which can be achieved by using this really cool gadget called the Galvanic Face Spa, sold through network marketing by Nuskin. I have gotten clients to use it with amazing results in just two months. It has different detachable "heads" that can be used for a five- minute face-lift, for wrinkles, or for the scalp. This device works on stimulating a deep circulation and lymphatic drainage by using micro-currents called galvanic currents, which the body cannot feel (so it does not create any sensation on the skin). Using this twice or thrice a week for five minutes a day is all that is needed.

» If you are looking for a supplement that can hasten this process, you can buy the company's Ageloc R2 product (that contains fermented cordyceps) that has been clinically proven to activate 'youth genes', and is mentioned in the *Physician's Desk Reference* (Doctor's Bible!), which is normally reserved for drugs.

Nails: These are a good indicator of nutrients in your body. If you have peeling nails, white marks, or chipping nails, this indicates poor/ lack of nutrients, especially B vitamins, zinc, and low trace minerals. If you have nail fungus, please note that it is always from the inside out: meaning you need to address the fungus internally as well as externally for permanent results.

Remedy: You can use essential oils like oregano, and apply on the nails externally. Internally, following an anti-candida protocol and detoxification are in order. An underactive thyroid may be indicated.

EAR, NOSE, THROAT, TONSILS:

» Once again, please use a lymphatic mover to clear the throat and tonsils of any infection or inflammation.

» Gargling with Himalayan pink salt and hot water morning and evening clears up even nasty throats.

» Using 15+ umf raw manuka honey, mixed with either turmeric powder, lemon/ clove/cinnamon essential oil (please use food-grade essential oils), or squeezed fresh ginger juice can work like magic to clear infection and inflammation rapidly. It tastes great too, so even fussy young ones will take it readily.

» Many a time, antibiotics don't work for sore throats, as these bugs have become antibiotic resistant, and sometimes the infection is a mix of virus and bacteria, so antibiotics won't completely do the trick. You can use diluted manuka honey with a little 30 ppm Argasol silver and water, and use a dropper for the nose and ears!

Upper Respiratory: This would be similar to ear, nose, and throat, and also follow instructions for clearing sinuses.

» The addition would be to use an ultrasonic essential oil diffuser in your room that can work deeper into your lungs to prevent the infection from moving to the lower respiratory system.

» Taking a few doses of liposomal vitamin C and vitamin D can boost immunity.

» I always recommend specific homeopathic remedies for infections that will clear it from the root.

Lower Respiratory: When you have a lower respiratory infection, it means it has reached the lungs, which is obviously not a good sign. This means your immunity is very low.

» You need to take all the supplements as mentioned in my supplement chapter, including a lymphatic mobilizer. What would immediately help in clearing up the infection is *not* a course of antibiotics—as such infections are almost always mixed with viral, bacterial, and fungal layers, even mycoplasma that add to the difficulty in clearing it up, that may be low grade, so not even detectable. Please use high-strength Argasol/Smart silver (*not* colloidal silver solutions).

» You should also diffuse and apply essential oils of hyssop, frankincense, eucalyptus, peppermint, ravensara, or any essential oil you may have—as they will still work to decrease infection and inflammation. They get to work almost instantly, as they don't need to be digested, but just breathed in, so keep them handy.

» If it is a stubborn infection like mycoplasma, please keep in mind that these bacteria-like organisms are much smaller than the average bacteria, and have no cell wall—so you cannot get rid of them with antibiotics. Antibiotics break open the bacterial cell wall causing the cell to effectively die. That's why mycoplasma is difficult to get rid of. There are very effective homeopathic mycoplasm remedies available through practitioners, so don't be disheartened.

HEART AND CIRCULATION:

» Please make sure that your dental checkups are up to date and you have replaced all metal fillings with ceramic ones (not your crowns, those are OK).

» Heavy metals greatly impact arteries and veins, disrupt heart functions, and can create heart arrhythmias.

» Do the heavy metal detox and use the basic supplements as mentioned. Liposomal vitamin C can improve results and inflammation markers.

» If your CrP protein is high (blood marker for high cardiac risk and inflammation), you need to further investigate the cause for this (it is toxicity related, but you need to identify the source, and nutrient deficiencies can make it worse). I find all clients who have the onset of a disease to be chronically and cellularly dehydrated.

» There are supplements like nitric oxide chewable called Circo2 that produce nitric oxide in the body that helps to relax blood vessels, improve cell oxygen, and blood flow. Athletes also take this to reap the same benefits to improve competitive edge.

» Some herbs that can be used (please check with a health care practitioner if you are taking medication, as there can be herb-drug interactions) are hawthorn, ginko biloba, L-arginine, and citrulline.

» Enzyme supplements like Neprinol/Cardio Enzymes or nattoki-nase help to *normalize* blood viscosity and even assist in reducing inflammation. These enzymes actually "eat up" or digest the plaque and residue on the arteries and can completely clear them up, no matter what your age.

» Women with heart palpitations and heart issues do need to work on hormone balance as well.

» Visceral fat loss can achieve a great leap in optimizing health in this area.

Digestive: This is too big of a topic, which is why I have dedicated an entire chapter to it. I would suggest everyone with any issues to get an advanced zyto scan done to assess for specific parasites, infections like candida, and get a zyto food scan done to identify food triggers that irritate the gut. Working on a customized protocol here is imperative in order to see lasting results. This is recommended for anyone with *any* chronic health issues.

Liver: Everyone can do with a liver cleanse, since we live in such a toxic world.

» If you want to address a fatty liver, you can absolutely reverse this serious condition by doing heavy metal chelation.

» If you are overweight, then doing the Ha2CG diet or the TR90 diet plan can get your liver enzymes back to normal. Many thyroid patients and smokers tend to get a fatty liver, and of course, very overweight people do as well. Do whatever it takes to get clean numbers, as the liver takes care of over 500 different functions in the body, and when it is compromised, it compromises all functions in turn. What would result are low immune responses, hormonal cancers, cardiovascular risks, and a host of other maladies.

» You can use milk thistle, dandelion root, MSM, glutathione, green tea, amino acids, zinc and other minerals, super greens like chlorella, antioxidant mix from super foods, and NAC (n-acetyl cysteine) all work (take a supplement like Thorne Research Mediclear Plus, or Youngevity Beyond Tangy Tangerine that has it all) in assisting the liver in a detox. **Note:** Please use a lymphatic cleanser along with a liver detox product, else you can be in trouble and feel worse off.

GALLBLADDER:

» Please ensure you are taking a vitamin D supplement at all times, as this reduces calcification and gall stone risk considerably. Please also read the section on cleansing the gallbladder.

» I like to work on meridian pathways when I see some stubborn situations. You can do acupuncture as the traditional method, but you can also use the DesBio Homeopathic remedies to work on these energetic pathways to get them "activated" again. This is user friendly for any age group, so it's my first choice.

» If you have your gallbladder removed, then you need to take an ox bile supplement with all your meals for the rest of your life, and definitely do the meridian activation once. A missing organ or system can put tremendous stress on other organs or systems, so correct support is essential. Acupuncture for this is also a good way to activate the meridian pathway.

Kidneys: The kidneys are the most delicate organ in the body. When there is organ failure, it is usually the kidneys that are affected first.

» If you are taking medications that can stress the kidneys, you need to work on the Kangen water and as much detoxification support as you can do for yourself.

» Using super greens like spirulina, aloe vera, potassium, zinc, turmeric parsley, and coriander are all beautiful at supporting the kidneys.

» Juicing or powders are the best way to use this.

» There are specific homeopathic detox drops available for kidney and bladder drainage that can be done.

» You need to do a heavy metal detox in order to get rid of them. They tend to "stick" to the detoxification organs like kidneys, liver etc.

Adrenals: There are many herbs that help improve adrenals. Most people don't know when they need to support their adrenals. I would almost always try and support adrenals, as long as we are aging and have stress to deal with.

» There are some beautiful herbs that can work like ginseng, Siberian ginseng, ashwagandha, cordyceps, and more. Remember that herbs can be like food, and may suit some and not others.

» The first primary support for adrenals would be to add pink Himalayan salt to one's diet. This alone can help prevent adrenal exhaustion, even during pregnancy.

» Another way to get around that is to use Apex Energetics adrenal cream application products or homeopathic adrenal support.

» You do need to identify low-grade infections and toxins/heavy metals and work on clearing them. They can stress adrenals and compromise the immune system.

» If you are an avid runner or have thyroid or sleep issues, then cortisol may be high or low. You do need homeopathic cortisol in order to balance that.

» Please try and avoid actual steroid hydrocortisone, as it can ruin your adrenal system completely. The best way to naturally help the adrenals is to rid your body of toxins, manage your stress, and sleep to recover.

Colon: The colon is also a large detoxification organ and needs to be cleansed regularly.

» The best way is to make sure you have at least two bowel movements a day, if not three. For a cleanse, please read the respective chapter. You can use Oxypower, a special kind of magnesium that cleans the colon by creating oxygen.

» Kangen water will do this in a similar way.

» Herbs like rhubarb, slippery elm, marshmallow, aloe vera, fiber like psyllium husk, vegetable fibers from all vegetables, and licorice root all support colon health.

» Most importantly, trace mineral supplements and staying hydrated can be excellent support for the colon.

» A colonic irrigation every once in a while can help to flush out accumulated toxins, as well as a salt water flush or taking liquids rich in enzymes.

Lymphatic: Most people don't have an idea of the lymphatic system. This is the first line of support that you would need to do when you are unwell, when undergoing any kind of a detox, for an effective weight loss strategy, or just to improve circulation, and prevent water retention.

» Unfortunately, there are very few good lymphatic cleansers, so only practitioner-grade ones make the cut. Desbio Bio Lymph phase, Desbio Lymphatic Drainage, or Metagenics Gtox Express works superbly well in this regard. Cleavers as an herb work really well, but I would use it with other herbs like in the Gtox Express.

» There are therapies like using a rebounder, a power plate, exercise, guasha (the Chinese art of scraping the body to improve blood flow), and the cupping method.

» Using the Nuskin Face/Body spa that can all be used to stimulate the lymphatic system.

Male Reproductive: Not much attention is given to the male reproductive system, except when there is a real problem.

» Ginsengs and cordyceps help with circulation, along with DHEA, and pregnenolone, a precursor to sex hormones that helps the body to convert it to whichever hormone it needs.

» Foods like maca, supergreens like spirulina, and phytoplankton are energizing and balancing, while herbs like tongkat ali, tribulus terrestris, and saw palmetto help improve hormone levels.

» Investigating the root cause(s) of low hormones is the real key, along with supporting and detoxifying the liver. If you are taking statins and your cholesterol is lower than 180 dl, it may be hampering your hormone production. Healthy cholesterol levels are essential, as cholesterol helps *produce* hormones.

» Celergen (mentioned below) can be used for male or female reproductive issues.

Note: Many men experience adrenal fatigue and are unaware of an underactive thyroid. Sport lovers need to be even more aware, especially those running marathons or in competitive sports.

Sperm Morphology: For healthy formation, sperm needs high nutrients like trace minerals of zinc, selenium along with B vitamins, amino acids, and antioxidants. Fertility drugs cannot improve sperm morphology. They may improve count, but nutrients are building blocks that create healthy sperm, so supplements are essential in turning around health.

Note: Almost always, heavy metal toxicity is involved; so get some professional help to assist you in clearing this.

Female Reproductive: There are some products that overlap and are gender neutral.

» Siberian ginseng and cordyceps work for females as well. Dong quai, red clover, red raspberry leaf, suma, maca, and other South American herbs from the Amazon help balance hormones.

» Pesticides, smoking, and chemical and heavy metal toxicities create endocrine/ reproductive imbalances. A detoxification program is essential in this regard.

» Visceral fat in excess can multiply hormone imbalances and create disease. Losing this fat will create health; either do the Ha2CG diet or the TR90 to assist in this regard. All the herbs and weight loss can assist in getting regular, healthy periods, improve fertility, and keep one looking and feeling young. Aging gracefully goes hand in hand with balanced hormones.

Teeth and Gums: This is a topic close to my heart, as I see many from toddlers to seniors struggle with maintaining healthy teeth. Our teeth are one of our most precious assets, as they really cannot be replaced. Nobody likes to go to the dentist. Hopefully by now you know to avoid fluoride in all ways. But to make sure you have good teeth, again, we need to know what teeth are made of.

» They are like external bone, so high amounts of calcium, boron, and at least 12 other minerals are required, along with amino acids, and gelatin to grow. So taking osteo Fx powder would be helpful.

» We also need healthy amounts of vitamin D3, so either getting 20 minutes of sun exposure daily, or taking vitamin D3 orally can help.

» We need to make sure the gums stay healthy as well. Taking a liposomal vitamin C, or nutrient dense super foods (high in vitamin C) can keep your mouth healthy.

» We also need to ensure that they don't get infected. Using essential oils in toothpaste like clove, peppermint, and wintergreen all reduce any inflammation and prevent any infection from setting in. They also indirectly nourish teeth. An amazing product worth mentioning here is from Ascended Health (USA). They have a product called Oralive, which uses edible clay, along with trace minerals, and essential oils that help healing, to nourish the gums and teeth and actually improve teeth/enamel density. You can swallow the "toothpaste" rather than spit it out, and it's good for health, too!

» Please note that it is from an acidic pH in the mouth from food remains along with bad bacteria that weakens teeth. If you have low stomach acid, or amalgam fillings, this can greatly affect the mouth pH, causing further rapid erosion of teeth enamel, even with great teeth hygiene.

» Flossing is an essential part of teeth hygiene, so teach your kids this invaluable habit.

» There are fascinating studies done on oil pulling–a centuries old custom in India. They use two teaspoons pure sesame or coconut oil to rinse the entire mouth for at least fifteen minutes, much like a mouthwash. This has shown to have a deeper and longer lasting cleansing effect in the mouth than even brushing! The amazing fact is, it seems to affect the entire body positively, not just the oral cavity. So this is one habit well worth pursuing!

Hair Loss for Males and Females: Hair loss for males has surprisingly similar reasons as for females.

» Hormonal imbalances

» Low zinc

» Poor circulation

» Low amino acids (protein blocks) which can be related to:

　　» Low stomach acid, low minerals especially iron

　　» Hormone disruptors or heavy metal toxicity

>> Underactive thyroid (subclinical: it does not reflect in a blood test)

Please read the relevant chapters to understand how you can support each of these underlying factors.

Early Greying of Hair: This is a result of low copper mineral in the body.

>> It can be reversed, not just by taking a chelated form of copper, but also by taking the synergistic 72 (plant based) trace minerals.

>> Even herbs like fermented cordyceps have helped people to sprout black hair, as it helps to revive adrenal function, and thus hormone balance, and circulation as well. Cordyceps are known to reactivate the youth gene clusters, similar to the prized ginseng.

Anti-Aging for Complete Well-Being: Since anti-aging is about staying young, looking young, and feeling young, there is one Rolls Royce of all supplements that come to mind:

>> Celergen, Swiss Cell Therapy. This is manufactured in Switzerland, is available in Asia as a supplement, and sold in the United States and Switzerland in anti-aging clinics and by aesthetic doctors. This is one supplement that currently has nothing else that is similar to it. It is based on fish DNA, using a cold extraction process that helps all cells in the body to detoxify, repair, and rejuvenate. It not only makes the person look younger, but also increases energy and libido, and works like a powerful anti-inflammatory.

>> Another product that has peer-reviewed research published on it is enzymes that increase telomere life in the body. The enzyme is called telomerase. It is now a well-known product, thanks to Hollywood. Suzanne Somers mentions it in her book, and network-marketing companies are using it in their supplements as well. Some

brand names are TA-65 and Telomerance.

» Another anti-aging supplement worth mentioning is one called Youth Span, created by Nuskin. It is a mixture of plant-based and essential fatty acids that works on activating at least six different sets of genes that keep one young and vital.

» Infiniti, a product by Juenesse Global, is a two capsule-twice a day supplement that works similar to Telomerase enzymes, but has other nutrients in it as well, like antioxidants, etc. Research has also shown that food-based resveratrol, found in berries like blueberries, grapes, raspberries, and mulberries, creates anti-aging effects similar to Telomerase.

» Immortalium, a product by Youngevity, was created for its anti-aging effects with similar ingredients as Infiniti.

Personally, I would go with supplements that enhance health, along with age, like Celergen. The simplest and most overlooked anti-aging nutrient was found after studies on the longest living cultures in the world were undertaken. The researchers found a common thread to their fantastic health: most lived close to glacier melts, which enrich their soil and water. These melts are extremely nutrient dense and high in trace minerals consumed by them. Remember, we are made from Mother Earth, and we need Earth's nutrients to keep us nourished in all respects. So minerals are the most basic supplement to keep all the metabolic gears well oiled and functioning.

Did You Know?

Maca, a turnip family vegetable found in South America, is an amazing energy boosting food that helps balance the entire endocrine system and all hormones? It has been taken for centuries as an aphrodisiac, as well as for endurance and stamina. It's also great taken in smoothies!

Two years back I was diagnosed with candida and lost 5kgs of weight in 3 months. I was underweight and my immunity was at an all time low. I tried to battle this problem with the help of my gynaecologist for one and a half years. My gynaecologist put all kinds of restriction on my diet and gave me loads of supplements, but could not help me with what I could actually eat. I have known Sheeba for over a year now but it never occurred to me that I should consult her or a nutritionist for my problem. Then, 4 months back I did consult Sheeba. Within a month my candida was gone, my immunity got better and I had gained 3kgs in 3 months.

I have spent thousands of dollars on GP"s, gynaecologists, and skin and hair doctors in the last two years to cure candida and the resulting ymptoms. Sheeba, with some supplements and proper diet plan cured my problem in just a month.

Anandi, 34, homemaker

CHAPTER 17

FAMILY FIRST AID AND TRAVEL KIT

This chapter is specifically for those who want to keep a few natural remedies at home that can save you the trouble of getting sicker or having to take strong medications. The same rules apply for your pets, but doses are considerably smaller. Also, most animals are extremely sensitive to smell, so make sure you diffuse essential oils they like, not run away from.

I always recommend practitioner-grade supplements for these emergencies, as they work quicker, and you can be sure of results. Generic brands just don't work as well. The very first supplements I would like to recommend are:

ALTERNATIVES TO ANTIBIOTICS:

» **SilverSolor Argasol/Smart Silver** (10vppm, 30vppm strength):

This is not colloidal silver, in that it goes through very high electric voltage of current and the liquid contains silver oxide. This is more potent than an antibiotic, as it stops bacteria, fungus, and virus dead in their tracks by preventing replication, and destroying their cell membrane. It does not affect good gut bacteria, which have a different 'electric charge' in comparison to the bad guys. This is extremely safe, even for babies, as its toxicity is as much as water! You need to have bucket loads of it for the body to show any toxicity. There are integrated doctors who give this as an IV instead of antibiotics. This would be the first line of defense for almost any kind of illness.

You need to use less of this than you would colloidal silver. If you don't have nano silver, then colloidal silver is fine, taken in larger amounts. You can make your own colloidal silver at home using a small device called "Silver Lungs." With this, you can make unlimited amounts at very low cost.

» **Green Brazilian Propolis**: Or any propolis, is a potent antiviral and antifungal. It is produced by bees to keep their hive germ free; it is also nutritive, and has quick healing powers when used. Especially good for sore throats, coughs, urinary tract infections, and any type of stubborn infection.

» **Grapefruit seed extract:** This is a bitter liquid, which makes it a powerful germicide. If you are not sure what kind of water you are getting, or are in an unclean environment where hygiene is questionable, it will "treat" the water and prevent any upset tummy. It can be taken as an alternative to antibiotics for any kind of infection.

» **Oregano Oil:** This is the most potent plant derived natural antibiotic. It is a powerful antiviral, antiseptic, antifungal, also used to relieve pain and inflammation, digestive, and respiratory issues, as well. This would be handy if your country had an outbreak of SARS, MERS, bird flu, etc.!

» **Olive Leaf Extract:** This liquid or capsule comes from the olive leaf. It is an amazing antiviral, antibacterial, and antifungal. If you were buying a retail supplement, I would recommend you take a bit more than the stipulated doses, and a little more frequently to see a shift in the infection. Can be given to kids but doesn't taste too good.

» **Venus Fly Trap:** This fly-trap carnivorous plant is a little healing miracle. The brand worth mentioning here is Carnivora, which has been clinically used for over 25 years. It has shown (in human and animal studies) to have immune modulating effects, and is used in autoimmune conditions, to treat tumors, is antiparasitic, antiviral, antibacterial, and antifungal. It is used in high doses in natural cancer therapy centers, and is a great weapon against all infections!

» **Garlic:** If there is no other item available, good old garlic is handy as an antibiotic. You can just slit the pod and swallow, or grind it and add it to raw honey and swallow. You can make a mixture with olive or coconut oil and apply to any infection or chest as a decongestant.

» **Lymphatic mover**: a strong lymphatic mover like echinacea, burdock, cleavers, or even Bio Lymphomyosot (practitioner homeopathic drops) get to work quickly to clear up congestion, phlegm, swollen lymph glands, and any type of infection. This would work equally well for a cough. Forget your cough syrups, as they are more harmful than helpful. Even detox teas with these ingredients are a nice gentle way to keep the lymph moving.

» **Therapeutic-grade Essential Oils:** These are extremely handy for cuts, bruises, headaches, cramps, stomach discomfort, any illness (antimicrobial, antifungal, antiviral, and anti-inflammatory), coughs, colds, and many more. There are many oils to choose from, but as a rule of thumb, make sure you have: Lemongrass, lavender, peppermint, eucalyptus, and clove cinnamon blend that can be either cold diffused (ultrasonically) or applied/rubbed directly onto the feet and ears. They create an immediate shift, but make sure to drink enough water.

» **Liposomal vitamin C:** This can be mixed in a drink or sipped to boost immunity instantly. It can work like a spring to bounce you back to health rapidly.

» **Vitamin D3:** Most people are low in this nutrient. Studies have found that people who stay sicker longer have much lower amounts of vitamin D in their blood than those who recover more quickly. Vitamin D is an immune booster and should be taken everyday. Adults can take 5,000 IU a day in general, and a little more when sick.

» **Vitamin A:** This is a very powerful immune booster. Take 10,000 to 20,000 IU of beta-carotene for three days, only when sick. This works like a jumpstart ignition.

» **Zinc:** An important nutrient to support immunity, many a times it comes in a blend with other immune booster herbs or supplements. Make sure it's an amino acid chelate. This should only be taken for a short duration. It is excellent, and a must if you have traveller's diarrhea, as it stops intestinal bacteria in its tracks.

» **Manuka 15+ UMF Honey:** This is a great wound healer and throat soother. I use it for cuts and wounds, any mouth ulcers, and even make sinus-clearing drops with it. It is also a great sore throat reliever. Just add a couple of drops of lemon essential oil (food-grade), along with some clove/cinnamon powder or oil, and mix with honey and just swallow a spoonful. Results are immediate. It has come back into mainstream medicine as a wound healer, and is called "medi-honey".

» **Probiotics:** These are especially handy if you have a stomach upset, or are on antibiotics. Take it for at least a few weeks or more. Keep it handy when travelling, as they are good for indigestion, constipation, or even traveler's diarrhea. A brand to mention here is Biogenics 16, a liquid bacterium with over 100 years of Japanese research. Bacteria and viruses mutate each year with the season, so flu shots just won't be effective. Best to avoid!

» **Iodine:** I would not go without this. As mentioned in earlier chapters, it is a potent immune booster and detox agent that helps oxygenate cells. Just a little every day is good immune support, so please don't take extra when you are sick, as it's not required.

» **Jet Lag:** Many days are wasted trying to adjust to time differences. It takes a toll on the trip as well as the body. I prefer to keep some supplement aid to assist the body gently with this process of adjustment. I love the homeopathies called Perfect Sleep (practitioner product), as well as the companion product called lunnasomm. Valerian, passionflower, and melatonin—all these may help to get your body to quickly adapt to the change and effect sleepiness. It needs to be used for a short period and is not habit forming. Perfect Sleep is great even for babies and children. Sleep inducing and calming teas are great. One great tip is, if you can plan to arrive at your destination when the sun is still out, go out and make sure you get some sunshine, as it plays a great role in normalizing your bio rhythmic clock. Keep busy in the day so hopefully sleep will not elude you in the night.

When traveling, I like to carry healthy food bars and single sachet packets of super greens and reds (mixed fruits and vegetables) that can help get you your healthy fix for the day, as you may not have much of a choice when it comes to food during travel.

Did You Know?

Goji berries are touted as a super food that is highly anti-aging? It is one of the most nutrient dense foods, and increases longevity, stamina, circulation, supports detoxification, and is excellent for eye health, and skin. Normally in premade marketed drinks, they are pasteurized (by law), and this lowers the nutrient levels, so having it in its original form is the best value for your money.

I have had a neurogenic bladder for decades. After surgery I was required to use a catheter 2-3 times a day, which brought on repeated urinary tract infections from time to time, especially when I travelled. This is the first time (ever) that my urine culture report had come absolutely clear, thanks to Sheeba's recommendations. Also, this was the first time I did not have to take antibiotics when I had an infection. For me, it was beyond my expectations. What docotors could not help me with, was solved in one session with Sheeba. recommend her to anyone who is looking for answers when there seem none.

I. B, 63, housewife

CHAPTER 18

HEALTH AND DISEASE MYTHS

Cholesterol: Did you know that there is no known disease linked with high cholesterol? Did you know that in the last few years, the high-end range was 220 dl and has now been further reduced to 200 dl?

Yes, you need to be concerned about the LDL, or the oxidized cholesterol, as that reflects damage. But high total cholesterol is not linked with heart disease. In fact, cholesterol is so precious that our liver produces it as a base for hormone production. So if you have less, you will experience (male and female) hormonal issues! Shockingly, low cholesterol dangers are many and real. It can range from depression, to all mental illnesses, hormonal issues, even schizophrenia. So is your statin helping you? Studies show that statins do not prevent heart attacks. Then why take them? Ask your doctor. They are selling more statins than before since the range was lowered. Lowering cholesterol has created a chronic ailment that did not exist fifty years ago—dementia. Dr. Joel Wallach's book *Dead Doctors Don't Lie* expounds on this. So do you need a drug to lower your cholesterol? No, but by following some of the detoxification protocols you can naturally bring it down—your healthy level may be 220 dl; another person's may be 190 dl. So don't get too rigid on the number factor.

Consuming dietary cholesterol (seafood, eggs, etc.), studies show, *does not* affect blood cholesterol. So save yourself the trouble! Also, please note, that it is a myth that any plant foods like coconuts and nuts have cholesterol in them! No plant foods contain cholesterol. You need to avoid refined and cooked oils that oxidize (like fried food), which increase LDL.

Hair Loss Drugs: Drugs prescribed to prevent hair loss actually dramatically reduce cholesterol as well, as the side effect may be fatty liver to boot. Now that we know we need to ensure our cholesterol does not dip too low, this drug is best avoided. Fatty liver is harder to reverse than low cholesterol, so find the solutions offered in this book for preventing hair loss, which work without the side effects.

Heatiness or Wind: Living in Asia, I get to hear this a lot. Many massage therapists will exclaim, "you've got a lot of wind". To a layman, this may sound rude, interpreting it as flatulence, but TCM practitioners refer to the "heatiness", or wind, as inflammation or stagnation. Which means, the wind can be anywhere in the body. Acupuncture or cupping may be recommended for this. My approach would be to get on an anti-inflammatory diet, work on detoxification, and do this every quarter or so, or layer the detoxification (there are many ways you can explore in the chapter on detox) from simple to slightly challenging. Anything that supports circulation, be it massage, exercise, or yoga, would support this process.

Exercise Makes Me Healthy: I have some very avid marathon runners and the like, who work out six days a week, have amazing bodies, and generally feel good. They even watch their diet to ensure the same. While this is wonderful, I have seen exactly such clients' blood test reports—shockingly poor. Surprised? They feel good and don't fall sick…so what's wrong? Being fit is not equivalent to being healthy. You may feel that way, as most get an adrenalin rush from running or with intense workouts. However, adrenalin increases the energy of your stress hormones at the end of the day. In fact, after a while, cortisol may be kicking in as well. If you keep triggering this hormone (which releases insulin for instant energy), it's like burning the candle at both ends, especially if you are not taking nourishing supplements that support build and repair in the body. Most such clients with this profile end up with hormonal issues, like adrenal fatigue, an underactive thyroid, varicose veins, etc.

HRT After Menopause: Don't be misguided by your doctors into taking HRT, especially if they are not bio-identical hormones. There is a world of a difference between synthetic and bio-identical (which are normally cream-based). If you really do have hormonal challenges, use the bio-identical ones, but do work on getting to the root cause of your challenges, as "old age" is definitely not a root cause. There are imbalances that cause this that need to be addressed. Osteoporosis and the like are all reversible, so do your homework on the right way to support your body. Traditional HRT is harmful, toxic, and now a known carcinogen…so *avoid* is the final word on that!

Birth Control Pills: Similar to HRT, synthetic hormones of any kind will ruin your entire body chemistry for any length of time taken. I have seen numerous clients who suffer terrible mood swings and hormonal challenges that leave them overweight, frustrated, and angry enough to stop the pill. What is the solution? Ideally, it should be the men who use the contraceptive, but if a woman really needs to, then of all the evils, the Mirena Ring is possibly the best option. Do not use copper IUD's as any metal, anywhere in the body creates further disruptions in overall health.

Fluoride For Teeth: Did you know that fluoride in our water supply and in dental procedures is making a zombie out of you? Fluoride was first introduced in World War II. It was sneaked into the enemy base camps water supply so they could weaken the enemy from the inside—it dumbs you down. It knocks out the iodine in the body that is required for immunity, hormones, metabolism, thyroid, and the brain. Exposure to chlorine does the same thing. Yes, even swimming or showering in chlorinated water causes absorption by the skin. You do need to use a good water and shower filter—and avoid fluoride treatments at the dentists!

Salt: Did you know that salt is actually good for you? Yes, even for those with hypertension. But what type of salt is important. Typical table salt is devoid and refined of all its original minerals (at least 72 different trace minerals are in sea salt). They add the iodine back as that is a governmental law, but not the rest of the 71 minerals. Is this harmful? Yes, this type of salt is harmful to the body, so avoiding it is wise. The type of salt you want to always include (and is good for you) in your daily cooking is not sea salt (which is white), as most sea salts are also bleached and treated. Original, unrefined salts are pink, grey, purple—any color rather than white.

So choose either Himalayan pink salt or Celtic Sea salt for your everyday cooking.

Protein Powders: Protein powders are over-hyped and over-used by all those who believe they need more protein because of their exercise. Yes, you do need the right proteins, without the junk in them. But, because you are what you absorb and not what you eat to a large degree, please avoid all protein powders which have long ingredient lists, especially those you can't pronounce. Most isolated proteins are not real foods, so those are to be absolutely avoided. Stick with few food-type ingredients. Some really good food-based proteins are Sun Warrior, Boku, Purium, and Garden of Life. Choose whole food-types that are sweetened with stevia and not artificial sweeteners or even fructose. Avoid slimming shakes that have too many foods in them, from super mushrooms, to goji berries, and exotic fruits. There is a 100 percent chance that there are a few ingredients among the many that your body may be reacting to (low grade sensitivity causing low grade inflammation). Please note that with any and all protein powders, your body needs to break it down to absorb it, and there is a higher stress on the kidneys and liver with increased consumption of proteins (especially for body builders). I do not recommend protein powders for athletes, but instead there is a safe and very effective solution. MAP or Master Amino Acid Proteins are tablets that are made purely from a specific patented sequence of amino acids that are absorbed into the blood stream in 23 minutes—so no "breakdown" by the body is required. This is good news, even for those with compromised digestion, like those suffering from auto-immune issues, cancer, and the like. It has next to nil negative effects or nitrogen waste, so it does not affect the kidneys or liver even with high doses, and therefore is a very safe protein supplement to take. I would recommend this for any age group—it should be based on their health condition, physical output, and body weight.

Hydrating Drinks: If you are one of those people who think it is "healthier" to consume these hydration drinks, then think again. It is unhealthy whether you are doing athletics or sweating it out. Smart athletes never put junk into their bodies—most hydrating drinks have high sugar content, along with flavorings and preservatives, and chemical names you can't pronounce. All of these add up to a big fat NO.

Instead, you get smart, nutritionally balanced drinks, meant for gamers and athletes under the Youngevity brand banner. Dr. Joel Wallach has created some drinks that pack a punch in terms of energy as well as nutrients.

If you aren't a big-time athlete, then keep it simple. Make your own. You can use coconut water with a pinch of Himalayan pink salt—it works better than any drink on the market.

If you don't have coconut water, you can use a little orange and lemon juice freshly squeezed, a little glucose, and pink salt. Dilute with water. This is very refreshing, even on a hot day or on a picnic.

Sunscreen Application: The media has driven fear into people that exposure to the sun without protection will cause skin cancer. I just want to make the facts clear. We are susceptible to *any* disease, only if internally we lack nutrients, hormones are off balance, have low antioxidants and cellular oxygenation, and so forth—repeated overexposure to the sun increases the propensity for skin cancer, but does not really cause skin cancer. Slightly different! In fact, healthy exposure to the sun is a must, and has amazing healing powers. We know that our body uses sunshine to make vitamin D, which in turn actually *prevents* cancer in the body. The sun also gives us energetic information that helps healing, similar to the earth (minerals).

It is actually more *dangerous* to use most of the sunscreens on the market. They have some of the strongest and most toxic chemical mixes—creating a dangerous synergy of chemicals that are actually carcinogenic! That is the irony.

So using sunscreens the smart way is my advice. It will prevent you from getting darker (notice I say darker, as it will not prevent you from getting dark—you will still tan, but not burn). Choose organic sunscreens that are safe and free from the nasty chemicals, and know that exposing your body to the sun for 20 to 30 minutes a day is actually very healthy.

Can't See, Can't Harm: EMF Blockers: Most people are aware of the proven negative effects of radiation from all computers and wireless devices, including radiation from just sitting on a plane. It would be wise to protect yourself from this unseen and insidious, ubiquitous exposure. It does distort energy and healthy vibrations, so make sure you use some electro-magnetic frequency blockers—there are many websites that sell stickers and such devices for cell phones, computers, large areas, homes and offices, as well as personal jewelry. Crystals like quartz and other semi-precious stones work in a similar way by emitting their own high vibrations and clearing negative frequencies; they are preferred by many healers in their work-spaces for this effect. EMF blockers would be great for pets as well, as animals are much more sensitive.

Did You Know?

Maqui berries are another superfood that is anti-aging, nutrient-dense, with high antioxidants? They have been eaten by the longest-living cultures in the world, and are a prized fruit due to their many health-giving properties.

I am a 32 yr female with a history of endometriosis and a failed IVF and I went to Sheeba after having undergone hormonal therapy, tried multiple other treatments which resulted in me feeling extremely tired, bloated and depressed without much remedy to the root problem. I did my own research and in the process tumbled upon Sheeba and just wanted to try her approach to healing. It has been 3 months for me into her regimen and I feel much better than I have ever felt in my life! I have almost no period clots and pains (which has been a lifelong event till now), my energy levels are back, I feel much more positive about life in general and the bloating and digestive issues are slowly disappearing too. I would recommend Sheeba to anyone who is looking to a holistic healing journey and if you thinking if you should make an appointment please do. You will not regret it."

D.C, Scientist, 32 yrs.

CHAPTER 19

NEW AGE THERAPIES VERSUS TRADITIONAL

Most people are wary and reluctant to try new therapies, modalities, and assessments. Many a time they have not found solace with the medical assessments and diagnostics, either. So to spend more money that is most likely not covered by insurance is wasteful. Having said that, there are many who are open to trying these modalities because they have not found answers to their health problems. It is important not to give up, and to keep asking questions, like, "What is the best way for my body to recover?" Sometimes the answer comes in surprising ways.

I would like to share my own story here. Due to an injury, I had developed spondylitis.

This was painful, limited my physical activity, and got me depressed, as physiotherapy was barely helping. I was open to trying anything in my desperation. I went for massages that gave temporary respite, and someone recommended a chiropractor. I went with no idea of what was about to happen, and after a lot of cracking, I found some relief, but I just couldn't get myself to go again, as I found the treatment very violent and forceful, and my body shuddered just thinking about it—it was a little like shock therapy to me. Somehow I understood that it was a great business model, but anything forced would eventually wind me up back to where I started. That's pretty much what happened, as I found my body had gone back to its painful contortion. The body has to be a willing participant to see sustainable results. Also, follow your gut instinct, and go back only if you are drawn to go again. The body will tell you what it wants and needs.

So I asked the universe, if not chiropractic treatment, then what?

I was working for an integrated wellness center then, and that week we had a very well known guest visiting. He was the foremost teacher of biodynamic cranio-sacral therapy. One session with him was like magic. There was an emotional, mental, and physical release that happened that propelled me to explore further. I attended several classes to learn, and to be worked on as well.

Needless to say, I got my spine back in place, and I was pain-free. In order to maintain that again, I asked, "What must I do?"

I started going for personal training to strengthen my back and core muscles. I still maintain this regime, and always listen to my body. At this point, I have to share that I did try one-on-one yoga, found that it felt good then, but then my back would get worse. Every time I went back to doing yoga, my back did not respond well. I got the same confirmation from some of my other clients with a similar back problem, who had also tried yoga to resolve it. I think yoga would help tremendously if done one-on-one in such situations rather than a group session.

So I decided to stick with personal training, which greatly improved my posture, and got my spine back in shape in less than two months. Each body is different, and however good the treatment may be, it may not be for you. Being able to discern what suits you may take time, and sometimes a health-care practitioner may give you the best advice as to what suits your condition so you don't have to go through trial and error.

Going back to talking about traditional systems of medicine. Systems like Ayurveda and Traditional Chinese Medicine (TCM) have been around for literally thousands of years. I believe in their diagnosis and holistic approach that assists in clearing meridians, energy pathways, and focuses on detoxification and supporting the digestive system as a first approach. Both systems focus on detoxification in different ways, and improving circulation. This approach would improve most people's conditions and they normally see improvement. Acupuncture, acupressure, herbal oil massages, cupping, etc. are all traditional ways of achieving this.

However, this system was established over 5,000 years ago, and is still valid today. But there are some missing links that these systems have not identified. All traditional systems do need an upgrade to fill in the gaps. Now we have doctors randomly prescribing antibiotics to all ages, even when a patient has a viral fever! The overuse of antibiotics was the start of gut dysbiosis and leaky gut, leading to allergies, and overgrowth of candida (fungus). This was not the case hundreds of years ago when there were no antibiotics. Another disturbing trend is that of heavy metal toxicity and multiple toxicity exposure from all personal care products and the environment. This creates a huge toxic load for the detoxification systems in the body, which most herbs can clear—but they do need to educate their patients that you need to avoid these toxins, else its back to square one. Another big issue is the multiple mercury amalgam fillings in teeth. It creates lifelong health challenges that may never resolve, unless a patient is made aware of it, and works on replacing fillings, and doing a heavy metal detox. It is a step-by-step, phase-by-phase process. Traditional systems are not able to identify such root issues for patients, so it may go unresolved for decades.

Another real concern now is that even the traditional systems of supplements or herbs can be sources of heavy toxicity. Many herbs come from China, where they are known to spray pesticides on them. The herbs are supposed to be stored in dark, cool jars, not in transparent glass jars that allow heat and light in. This destroys the basic properties of the herbs. They were originally stored in wooden chests of drawers for that reason. So even traditional systems have moved away from the traditional systems! Ayurveda is known to use heavy metals in some of their tonics, as it is part of the protocol. I don't know if it really helps or not, but I personally wouldn't take herbs laced with pesticides or heavy metals.

If you know you are using organic herbs that have a standardized strength, that are well preserved (in capsules or in a liquid gel cap), then that would be a safer or more sensible option.

If you choose to see a modern doctor, then choose an integrated doctor who can treat you with natural remedies alongside medications you may need. These medical practitioners are normally open to reducing medication doses or helping you to wean off it completely, depending on your progress.

Let's talk about New Age Therapies now. I believe that all these new therapies are not really new—they actually follow ancient laws and systems that are now available in an easy to use format for the masses!

Here are a number of therapies (old and new) that can assist in deeper and more permanent healing. Remember that you want to have a pattern that combines the physical aspect for detoxification and increased circulation, using a method below, eg., Far infrared sauna. Along with this, use a method that can address emotional and mental issues, for example, Bach flower remedies and one or two sessions that work on things unseen in the fifth dimension, like, reconnected healing.

I am going to touch upon some therapies here, and if you are keen to know more, please check in the resources section, where you can find more information on each.

Hyperbaric Oxygen: This therapy is normally available in an integrated doctor's clinic. It uses oxygen in a pressurized environment that speeds up healing processes in the body, and can be used for any health issue. Please see resources for details. This is a natural alternative to a lot of toxic medication, including radiation and chemotherapy, antibiotics, etc. This is very useful for someone with chronic or recurring illness, cancer, athletes who need quick recovery time, or an elderly person who cannot tolerate drugs well, or has a weakened immune system. Before lungs fill up with water and there is hospitalization required, hyperbaric oxygen can actually save a person's life.

UVB Phototherapy: This is ultraviolet light therapy that works effectively on psoriasis and similar skin conditions. It is normally under a medical setting, and is not a medication or drug, so most are happy to try this for their condition. It can be done at home, but the equipment needs to be medically prescribed.

Ozone: This therapy introduces oxygen in the body using ozone. There are many ways this could be administered—air via rectal, IV infusion, or in the blood via auto-hemotherapy (blood taken out, charged with ozone, and then re-injected into the patient). It enhances stamina, endurance, rapidly clears any infection in the body, works as a super-antioxidant, reduces inflammation, and more. Who should consider it? Anyone with chronic health issues or pain.

Light Spectrochrome: This might be the most cost-effective and least-involved treatment you can do for yourself or your loved one.

Different colors of light have different wavelengths that create healing in the body. This is a very old science known as color therapy. You can create medicinal water and simple medicines based on this—the book I would recommend is *Let There Be Light*. It can help with a range of issues like healing severe burns, absorption of nutrition, circulation, infections, poor sleep, fibromyalgia, old age infirmities, asthma, arthritis, pain, etc.

Stem Cell: Another controversial therapy is stem cell, and there are a few versions of this. The relatively safer approach is the stem cells taken from your own body fat cells, which are extracted and activated in the lab and then pumped back into your body intravenously, and via injection on specific spots. I have personally seen remarkable transformation in patients—cured and youthful are the words you can use. This therapy applies to anti-aging, cancer, AIDS, autoimmune, and any ailment under the sun. The long-term repercussions to this therapy are yet unknown. After the stem cell therapy, if you continue living the same lifestyle as you did before you had cancer, will the cancer eventually come back? Most likely; however, there hasn't been any studies done that follow patients after their treatment.

Prolozone: Prolozone® is a homeopathic/oxygen-ozone injection technique developed by Dr. Frank Shallenberger. It is excellent for all forms of musculo-skeletal and joint pain, including chronic neck and back pain, rotator cuff injuries, degenerative and arthritic hips and knees, degenerated discs, and shoulder and elbow pain. Because in many cases Prolozone actually corrects the pathology of the disorder, there is a 75 percent chance for the chronic pain sufferer to become permanently pain free. Prolozone is a form of non-surgical ligament reconstruction, and is a permanent treatment for chronic pain. Prolozone is a connective tissue injection therapy of collagen producing substances and ozone gas, which can reconstruct damaged or weakened connective tissue in and around joints. These substances are injected into the damaged connective tissue in and around a joint to rebuild the damaged areas.

DEVICES:

EMF blockers: I would always use electromagnetic frequency blockers—there are many different types available on the Internet, ranging from stickers to blocks to jewelry…whatever works for you. Use them everyday, especially when you are travelling on a plane. Nowadays, with everything being wireless, we may not have a mobile phone on us, but we are still exposed to the radiation—kind of like passive smoking. It's all around us. Connecting with nature is now more important than ever before for this very reason. Do it regularly in any manner—it could even be as simple as sun gazing for five minutes in the morning.

Rife Machine: This is a small tape recorder-sized device that has been around for decades. Why don't you know about it? Well, you are not *meant* to know about it.

It is a frequency zapper of sorts—it literally zaps frequencies of virus, bacteria, parasites, fungus, and tumors from your system. This sounds simple enough, but the repercussions to that are enormous! Almost all chronic disease states are related to insidious infections, and when they finally start to clear, they can eradicate the disease itself. It has helped people all over the world get rid of cancer, diabetes, pain, parasitic infections, etc. I would recommend getting the JWLABS brand, as there are many kinds of Rife machines around. This one has a good track record and 24/7 customer support.

Vielight: This intranasal, non-invasive photo-light device originally developed in Russia, and has sold over 10,000,000 units all over the world. It is a very simple light that gets clipped onto your nose and works on the dense blood capillary network just under the sinuses. It boosts the immune system, lowers blood pressure, improves metabolism, and reduces insomnia, allergic rhinitis, and sinus issues without any side effects. And yes! It can be used for children of all ages as well. This phototherapy works across numerous cellular mechanisms of action to achieve its profound therapeutic effects. It improves cellular oxygenation, blood lipid balance, and even helps those with Alzheimer's and Parkinson's. It is also a veritable anti-aging tool, as it acts like a potent antioxidant.

Physical Therapies: There are many physical therapies that can assist in healing the body.

Body works: This is under the physical therapies category, normally using physical touch.

Massages: The most basic is massage. There are many types of massages to explore: Sport, Chinese meridian massage, aromatherapy, including many styles of massage. All massages help to improve circulation, some being specific for injuries.

For specific back issues like misalignment, there are some that may benefit:

Pet therapy: Never underestimate a friend, especially the four-legged kind. They provide unconditional love and heal in their own way. They also bring joy to a home, these little pleasures being more significant than any other physical therapy.

Pets are now being used in hospital wards and old age homes for this reason.

Bowen therapy: This is a gentle touch therapy that helps the body/muscles to break old patterns and register new patterns, so alignment can happen gently. It can be a little strange for someone doing it for the first time, as the practitioner will leave the room from time to time during a session to let the body rest and integrate.

Chiropractic adjustments: This is a popular form of bodywork, more specific for the spine, to help it align. Many people benefit from this treatment, but need to go to quite a few sessions to gain results. The adjustments are gentle, but still forced. I personally find it a great business model for the chiropractors, but not a solution-based therapy for the patient. When something is forced, the body fights back and autocorrects to the old pattern. Hence, you need to go for regular adjustments. There are definitely other therapies out there that need to be done only a few times to reap benefits, unlike chiropractic. I would personally avoid this form of treatment as benefits may or may not last.

Biodynamic Craniosacral Therapy: This therapy is very gentle and healing, whose workings are based on quantum physics. It is a light touch along the spine and head that applies no pressure or force. It is considered a meditative therapy that works on switching off the sympathetic system (the stress system) and instead switches on the parasympathetic response in the body (the relaxed state). In this state, the body rejuvenates, reorients, and heals. Most clients fall asleep within the first 10 minutes of the session, but a conscious, meditative state of sleep where they are aware of their environment. It helps to release body tightness and compression that unfolds and releases stored emotions and memories as well, so it works deeper than just the physical level.

Auriculotherapy: This therapy is basically acupressure or acupuncture, using reflexology points all along the ears! So it's working within the small space all along the ears that makes it quick and painless that has shown to have 95 percent efficacy in helping quit smoking! It can be used for any pain or weight gain—it brings the body to balance. I highly recommend this therapy as the quickest and surest way to support your body and goals.

Quantum Touch: This method uses a breath technique and some simple hand positions on the client either physically, or remotely. It is a simple, yet effective technique in quantum resonance—increasing the frequency of the practitioner and client, which then clears the body of lower-lying vibrations like pain, infections, and other ailments. There are amazing success stories, and it can be learned by anyone—even little children, who are especially good at it!

NAET (Namboodiripad Allergy Elimination Technique): This was also founded by a former chiropractor, Dr. Devi Namboodiripad. It is a technique that works on the spine and breathing to reduce or remove allergy patterns in the body. Many have had lifetime allergies removed by using this technique. I personally have used it, but did not see any results for my rhinitis, and had clients report they did not have much success with it either. I would not write it off, as many integrated doctors in the United States have found it useful. I find that results may vary depending on the practitioner. When combined with specific NAET homeopathic formulas, the therapy is that much more effective.

Sound Therapies: This includes things like the tuning fork, Tibetan Bowl, and chanting, and are beautiful, uplifting ways to change your biochemistry instantly! It works to switch off stress and switch on happy neurotransmitters, and actually rewires the brain! This can be done as a daily practice. Just listening to the right or healing frequencies can be their own complete therapy.

Energetic Therapies: Reiki is the most popular energy-healing modality, along with Pranic healing. It is a channeling of universal life force energy from practitioner to receiver. There have been many healing testimonials, as these are centuries-old practices. None of these healing modalities have anything to do with religion.

Quantum Healing or Fifth-dimensional Healing: There are many out there who are at a higher state of vibration, who can help to change your vibrational state in an instant. We actually do have the privilege of having advanced beings on this planet, who help to shape our destiny of human consciousness. There are many light workers, but getting to know even one who is the "real deal" versus a sham can be tricky. A light worker is someone who has unmasked the veil of the three-dimensional world, and can see/interact with energy and subtle dimensions. This could mean spirits (like angels, not ghosts!) in the subtle realm, or just unplugging from the three-dimensional grid system we are all plugged into, to create healing that can only be explained by quantum physics.

Reconnective Healing: This falls under the category of fifth-dimensional healing. It is not energy healing, and it goes beyond techniques. You can read about it in Dr. Eric Pearl's book, *The Reconnection.* I was so fascinated by his book that I attended his seminar, and became a reconnective practitioner. You can read more about spontaneous healings in Gregg Braden's book, *The Spontaneous Healing of Belief.*

If you are interested in working with a light worker, please see the resources section of this book. For those who are skeptics, or just not ready for this, I did warn you that you needed to keep an open mind while reading this book!

Star Healing/Intergalactic Healing: This is a fifth-dimensional, very new (as of 2011) healing that has been channeled by Kelly Hampton, that works with the Pleiades constellation and star energies, that have been experienced as very powerful and almost miraculous. Typically only one 60 -minute session is required, and can be done remotely.

Aura Soma/Color Therapy: This falls under the fifth-dimensional category of healing as well. It is a beautiful, almost visually stunning system of intuitively choosing colored bottles that are made with plant energies, crystal, light, and love. This therapy works on all dimensions of energy, including our auric field, our energy bodies, and chakras, as well as connections with higher-energy bodies. This can be used on children and adults. My own experience with this has been amazing. My son had the habit of biting his nails ever since he was four years old. The weird thing was that he also bit his toenails! I had not cut his nails in over six years. After using the aura soma–chosen bottle, he stopped biting his nails completely! Certain insecurities and emotions that are invisible are taken care of by this fascinating therapy.

Brain and Body Regeneration: This may come as a shock to most, but there are people who are already re-growing body parts, including the brain. No sci-fi, no lab—just using the quantum field. The stranger-than-fiction part is that they are teaching anyone and everyone who wants to learn to do it too! Some well-documented people you can Google are Julie Renee Doering, who has regrown people's colons (surgically removed), repaired brain-damaged individuals (due to accidents), and regrown thyroid, adrenals, etc., including her own.

Dr. B. M. Hegde is an award-winning doctor who has proven to the medical world that it can be done without any fancy science or technology. The power of intention and thought is the basis for this magic.

I was reading *Harry Potter*, where they can regrow bone and flesh, and thought that was really cool. But this magic is for real.

So if you are in a situation where a body part has been removed, you can choose to regrow it. Or, better yet, if you have a poorly working body system, you can choose to repair all of it. Each cell in our body is in itself a complete blueprint or hologram that can be used as the basis to generate any other cell in the body. But it is done with intention, not in a lab. I would like the readers to explore and research this on their own, as this topic warrants that. It is eye opening and one would wonder why no one has heard of it, why it's not in some Guiness world record book, or why doctors are not excitedly discussing the immense possibilities.

This quantum healing can be used for any type of healing—disease of any kind, not just regeneration. It can even be used for spiritual growth.

There are *many* other healers that are under this category of quantum healing. They can activate change in the body by altering or increasing the body's resonant frequencies. For we all know that our own vibration or resonance, e.g., mindset of "money is evil"—will not be able to attract abundance. When this frequency changes to: "money is a tool I can use it to help people," it attracts the energy of money, and the person's abundance shifts. Since everything is energy, when we work on that, the outcomes change, and our reality shifts.

The most empowering aspect is that it can be learned by anyone, and kids are better at it than adults!

Please see the Appendix for a list of healers who work in this area.

Scientifically Proven Therapies for Cancer: There are more cases of cancer than ever before. We all know someone suffering from it. This information may help to save their lives and prevent suffering. Information is power, and opens the door to choices. Did you know that collated studies have found that for adult onset cancers (any cancer), chemotherapy is 98 percent *ineffective?* That is jaw-dropping information. That means chemotherapy is not based on *any science at all.*

Then why is everyone doing it? Let's just say it's a multibillion-dollar industry. Do your research. It's all out there. Poisoning our bodies to get rid of the cancer is like bombing your house down to get rid of a spider. Why and how do people survive after chemotherapy? We underestimate our bodies' powers of rejuvenation. We also underestimate our will and spirit, as amazing human beings. It is this that keeps us going, despite the poisons.

Some saner and healthier, immune-supportive, scientific cancer protocols are:

Low-dose Insulin Potentiation Therapy: This is chemotherapy at very low doses, along with insulin that works like a heat-seeking missile targeting cancer cells. So very little drug is required to make the difference, while preventing the devastating side effects of standard chemotherapy by up to 95 percent!

Gc Protein-derived Macrophage Activating Factor (GcMAF): These are immune cells we all have that get suppressed when a person has cancer. In this case, these killer cells are introduced via intra muscular injections that boost the immune system and eliminate cancer cells rapidly. The success rate for cancer and autism is an astonishing 80 percent! They are manufactured in Europe.

Hyperthermia: This treatment for cancer exposes the body to high temperatures of up to 45 degrees Celsius that damage and kill cancer cells, with minimal injury to normal tissue. Cancer cells are more sensitive to high heat. Using this as an advantage, hyperthermia can shrink tumors rapidly.

IV Drop Vitamin C, Sodium Selenite, and B17: These vitamins are given intravenously that work as instant antioxidant nutrients, while the B17 and sodium selenite selectively kill only cancer cells.

Ozone therapy: This works by extracting your own blood (100ml to 500ml) and then infusing it with ozone and reintroducing this highly oxygenated blood back into your body via IV; this has been done legally for decades by athletes to boost their endurance.

Such therapies and treatments are mostly covered by insurance (especially if oncologists or qualified medical doctors are working with you), so they would be a first-line defense choice for someone with cancer. These therapies are available in Bangkok, Thailand at the Veritalife Centre, in Spain at the Budwig Cancer Center, Mexico, parts of the United States, many places in Germany, Switzerland, and around Europe, who are main supporters and researchers of natural therapies.

Please note that some therapies mentioned here, like vitamin C and ozone IV, hyperthermia, assisted lymph drainage, and colonics can all be done as a clinical detox—even when a person is healthy. It is my first choice recommendation, rather than going to a health resort. Veritalife Healthcare Centre in Bangkok offers it, along with Budwig Centre in Spain. Other cancer centers around the world that have these programs should be able to accommodate requests for short clinical detoxes as well.

> **Did you know?**
>
> Vitamin D can slash cancer risk by 77 percent? But the scary news is that most people are severely deficient in vitamin D, and RDA levels are not sufficient to prevent cancer.

I went to Sheeba on end August 2014. I am 37 years old guy with 187cm height and 106kg weight, I was also having high blood pressure (for last 5 years) and was in the preliminary stage of diabetes. Although I am not a great foodie, i am bit of an emotional eater and doesn't have much control especially in occasions or when having some delicious dishes. The thing I liked about Sheeba is that she diagnosed every minute details in my blood report and even checked whether I have any filling in tooth or not. After going thru her diet course along with the supplements, I am now having 93Kg of weight with much less fat percentage, increased muscle mass and reduced visceral fat and the entire process took exactly 4 months. I can't remember the last time when i had this kind of figures. I am grateful to Sheeba for letting me know to understand my body which I believe is the greatest gift in new year 2015. I believe in long term result and I now have normal blood pressure, blood sugar and my uric acid numbers have reduced along with my fatty liver.

The only drawback is : my wife is complaining that she is losing her wardrobe space to accommodate my new trousers and shirts."

S.M, Mechanical Engineer

CHAPTER 20

FEELING GOOD AND LOOKING GOOD

have many people come to me for vanity's sake. They have skin challenges or just want a better figure—they are all valid reasons to not looking good—but good nutrition makes you *feel* good too. That is the happy side effect. For best results, we need to target two areas: internal and external.

Inner to outer:

The face reflects the internal systems, just like reflexology. If you have eye bags that start to reveal themselves, it's not because you are getting old, but because your kidney and liver are not detoxifying as they should.

We all believe in sending our cars in for regular maintenance; the same rules apply to us. We need tune-ups and maybe even continuous support to ensure our systems are running at optimal. There are many approaches on how to do that, but the detox chapter is useful in getting a feel of where to start.

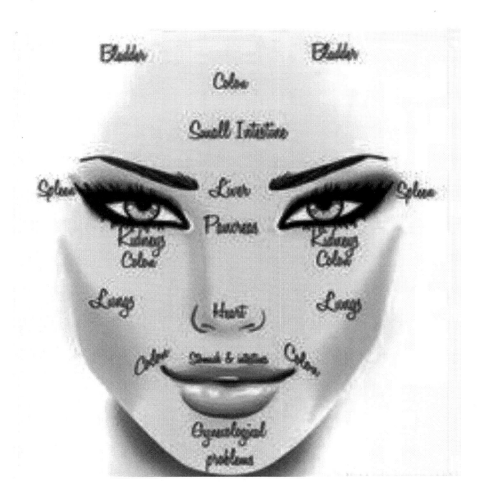

My recommended approach for adults would be:

1) Start with a blood test to discover any nutrient highs/lows/imbalances

2) Plug in these gaps by taking professionally advised nutrients

3) Support the body with some form of detoxification—that could be homeopathic, diet alone, herbs, vitamins and nutrients, or physical therapies like far infrared sauna or some healing modality that can raise your vibrations.

4) Some permanent lifestyle change(s) that makes sense to you at that point: it could be as simple as praying or blessing your food before eating it.

5) Physical or external ways, like applying effective serum or cream on the face to improve elasticity or texture of the skin.

PHYSICAL OR EXTERNAL APPLICATIONS:

I do have my personal favorites in this category. As a woman, I believe in presenting myself in the best light, and practicing what I preach.

Some tried and recommended products are:

Must have: I love the Nuskin Face spa. I stopped going for facials, and instead use this handheld device for five minutes a couple of times a week; this completely transformed my face to a younger version of me. These results are permanent, not cosmetic. The face spa is a patented device using galvanic (micro) currents that stimulate the lymphatic and deeper circulation to the whole face, creating instead a deep therapeutic massage-like effect, while the gels help to deep clean the skin. The treatment lasts for all of five minutes, and you can see the difference immediately after! It's like someone ironed out your face, giving it more lift and contour, and making it visibly cleaner and brighter. Products you apply after the treatment will have 80 percent more effectiveness. So that takes us to what to apply after.

Applications: Nuskin has their own anti-aging paraben free Ageloc serums and creams that work well. There are many networking companies that sell really good organic skin care.

I don't necessarily think organic skincare is better or more effective—I find the opposite to be true. There are some skin care products that are not organic, but are free from the chemicals like Luminescence adult stem cell products. They use growth factors extracted from stem cells taken from adult fat cells. Stem cells are another hot topic that is very promising, but still a little controversial as a therapy. This serum has shown remarkable healing and rejuvenating abilities that create some amazing before and after pictures and stories.

(See appendix on how to order)

I also believe that since we do need to supplement our diet, similarly, we need to use vitamins for our skin.

I would recommend a 22 percent vitamin C serum (liposomal delivery form), along with a mixture of vitamin E, and you can layer a moisturizer that contains some vitamin A, and a water-based UVA/UVB blocker.

I recommend some gentle exfoliators that feel like toothpaste or gel rather than gritty—please do not abuse your skin with gritty cleansers. Such cleansers can harm skin and are never recommended.

I also like night creams that have some element to improve elasticity—mentioned in peer-reviewed medical journals and well researched ingredients like Equol. The company name using this product is called YU Infini serum. It helps to reduce the aging hormones on the skin while improving elasticity and texture by over 90 percent! That is impressive science, unlike the clinical studies you hear of being done by skin care companies in-house.

Body skin care: There are many who have to experience winter every year. We all know that the skin dries up; it's a challenge to stay moisturized and maintain good skin during these months. This is especially evident for those with skin concerns like psoriasis, etc. I advise my clients to stop using soap bars during this time. Organic body gels and scrubs are preferable, as they are not as alkaline and drying. The other option I love is to make my own nourishing scrub. Just use pink Himalayan salt and add either extra virgin olive oil, coconut oil, or food-grade Argon oil, and scrub on body.

Then, simply rinse off. Not only will it clean and exfoliate well, but it also hydrates the body and locks in the moisture. You will find you may not even need a moisturizer afterwards. If you don't care for the smell of the oil, add some essential oil that you like to keep it pleasant smelling.

DARK EYE CIRCLES AND EYE BAGS:

I have many clients who rightly infer that they may have nutritional challenges when they start to get dark circles or under eye bags. This is not a hereditary condition, and is directly related to your organs and detoxification systems (see face diagram).

Causative factors:

» Dark circles generally mean you are lacking essential minerals that are required by all cells, specifically the kidneys and liver. The organs use these nutrients as tools to continue their detoxification work. When in short supply, congestion or stagnation of these organs is reflected in the delicate eye area.

» Sometimes clients may be low in iron as well; a blood test is the best way to screen for this.

» I also find that even if the client has regular bowel movements, it does not mean that it is good enough. Everyone ideally needs to have two to three bowel movements a day. Large intestine congestion is also indicated.

» Most clients also have heavy metal toxicity. Please read the heavy metal detox chapter to clear your body of these.

» Sometimes clients taking medication have multiple side effects, so this could be a causative factor as well.

» Capillary congestion (circulation) along with inflammation related to the above points

Almost always, people with eye bags and dark circles have cellular dehydration, for which please read my chapter on water and correct hydration.

So far, three things need to be done internally:

1. Optimize cellular hydration
2. Optimize minerals including iron check
3. Support detoxification systems through homeopathy or nutraceuticals

We also need to do some external support to get this into the fast track. The capillaries and circulation under eyes are poor, and just like a body massage, need some regular stimulation to improve.

The best way to see results (especially for eye bags) is to use the Nuskin Face spa mentioned earlier. If you would like something more cosmetic, i.e., short-lived, then the Ageless product by Jeunesse works in seconds to reduce eye bags. The effects last for about eight hours, after which it gets back to the original puffiness.

As I write this book, Juenesse has come up with an eye-firming gel that works on permanently reducing eye bags and dark circles, based on Dr. Nathan Newman's work. This would be a must try!

Body Shaping and Cellulite: Of course the natural way is the best way—by that I mean without the use of fancy aesthetic equipment that re-contours your body.

Personal training to tone and strengthen muscles can get you healthy and fit. Another easily doable recommendation is to join a gym that has a Power Plate machine. This is a vibrato machine (I am specific about the brand Power Plate, not just any vibrator machine). Simple exercises on this can strengthen and tone the body—15 minutes on this machine is equivalent to a 45-minute workout. Even an 80 year old can use it and benefit.

If you want to specifically work on stubborn areas like thighs, arms, etc., then you can use the home use Nuskin body spa. This is a stronger version of the face spa, which conducts galvanic currents to the skin, which then penetrate and stimulate circulation and lymph—a deeper penetration than any type of massage can induce. If you are able to use this regularly (at least thrice a week), the results are visible. They are especially good for those with cellulite, for lifting bust and butt. It is the best available DIY system in the privacy of your own home.

One thing that I have to mention, is that many women get manicures and pedicures—while it's nice to have well-manicured nails, please choose to do it with organic, hormone-disruptor-free nail varnish. Other chemicals are harmful to the applier and the wearer—there are many articles on this in the news, so listen well! If you love nail varnish, you can choose healthier ones that will not disrupt your hormonal balance.

I am 32 years old female with 155cm height and 64kg weight. Since the birth of my first child I became really overweight and was diagnosed with high blood pressure . I was prescribed to have pressure medications everyday for the last 6 years by my cardiologist in Singapore. I tried all kinds of exercise and diet to lose weight but nothing seemed to work; this often left me feeling frustrated and depressed. In fact, recently my health really deteriorated; my blood pressure started to fluctuate and my blood reports showed high levels of blood sugar, cholesterol, and tri glycerides. That's when my cardiologist recommended me to go to Sheeba to and see if her diet could help to reduce some weight. I used to struggle even to lose one or two kilos in the last few years so never thought any diet could ever help me reduce substantial amount of weight.

I went to Sheeba in November 2014. And she was a MIRACLE!!!!

Please note that despite the fact that I do not live in Singapore, Sheeba managed to transform my health!

Sheeba's diet along with the supplements she prescribed helped me actually lose 10 kilos in a span of 3 months . Now I weigh 54 kg and I can't remember the last time when I weighed so less . The thing I liked about Sheeba is that she diagnosed every details in my blood report and based on that recommended a diet. Now all my blood pressure and all my blood reports have become normal . The best part is that, with my pressure becoming normal , my doctor got me to stop my medication.

I feel so much more confident now. I am the fittest I have ever been and I am really grateful to Sheeba for helping me to adopt a healthy lifestyle. I would recommend Sheeba to anybody who wants to get back to shape.

Karina. I, 32yrs, Housewife

CHAPTER 21

SPIRITUAL NUTRITION

This topic is very close to my heart, as it deals with everything else that no one wants to address, and is not in the physical realm of nutrition and well-being, yet it is probably the most powerful and life-changing tool once accepted and utilized.

I am talking about the unseen energy that is present everywhere. If we work on ourselves by eating healthier, exercising, and becoming positive-minded, then we have covered mind-body only. What about spirit?

If we are nourishing ourselves, we need to make sure that the space we dwell in is equally harmonious for healing to happen. It's like taking a bath and then swimming in the mud. You would need repeated baths to stay clean!

So make sure your work and home spaces are high in good vibrations. Feng shui is a popular method in the east, but in line with keeping things simple and cost-effective, my favorite is Mashhur Anam's Holographic

Feng Shui, offered online for a few hundred dollars (and not the few thousand you would spend on restructuring your house/items). This can work on all negative lines, energies, and harmonize all spaces with the individuals living in the space, based on the zodiac sign for the year, e.g., Year of the Wooden Horse.

This kind of complete energy work on the home can create healing, abundance, prosperity, peace, joy, and a sense of wellbeing to all people who reside in or enter that home.

The other way to improve the vibration of the home is to use Kelly Hampton's *Ascended Spaces* guidebook on a more DIY approach.

Another aspect is that, believe it or not, there may actually be energy entities or spirits who are residing in your body or home without your permission. Many energy healers have seen this, and have had to address it to allow complete healing to happen. Remember that we are light beings and entities are attracted to the light.

I am not talking about demonic possessions or wild spirits here, just spirits who have not moved on, or even a loved one you have not let go of. You do need a practitioner who does energy work, as it cannot be done on your own. There are a few practitioners I would recommend: Mas Sajady, Julie–Renee Doering, Jarrad Hewett, Kelly Hampton, and Mashhur Anam, who can all work on you remotely. Please check the appendix for their websites.

Another aspect of spirit is well addressed by Caroline Myss in her book, *Anatomy of the Spirit*. She gives some beautiful examples of how when the emotions heal, the body heals itself, and no further intervention is required. An example of this would be the true story told by my meditation teacher, Drunvalo Malchizedek. An old friend approached him and requested healing; this woman had terminal cancer, with only weeks to live.

In his meditation, however, he was told not to do any healing. Instead, he was given specific instructions on how he could help her. He went to her after having bought a teddy bear and a closed bud rose, with a piece of paper with some words written on it, as he was advised. She received it with a little surprise and thanked him. But the moment she read the note, she burst into uncontrollable sobs. He left her to deal with her grief privately. In the months that followed, she finally contacted him to let him know that she had completely recovered (with no sign of cancer), and was doing very well. She shared that all the items he had given her were the last few things her dad had given her as a little girl before he passed away. She had held that trauma of his death in her cells. When she released that trauma and allowed herself to let it go, it released her toxic/bottled emotions, which then allowed her complete recovery.

This sounds like a fairytale story, but there are many people and many different stories like these. Every single one of our cells in our body responds to emotions, both positive and negative—a moment of awareness can create a miracle. Sometimes we need healers and practitioners who can reflect this to us, to create the awareness where we never thought to look, thought we had "dealt" with, or may have been so young (or even as a fetus) that we did not even have a recollection of the trauma.

Life is a journey, and I believe we need to continue to evolve, and seek people, ideas, and technology that can help further that.

If you have chronic pain, infections, repeated falls, fractures, and imbalances in many areas of your life other than nutrition, seek help with such practitioners who can go deeper and work on you. My own experience has been that not just health, *but all aspects and areas of life improve*, as they are all linked to certain root emotions or energy stagnations.

A point to note here: I have clients who have done a lot of energy work, or meditate and feel they are evolved souls. They come to see me for various health reasons. I always find that we need to work on our spirit, yes, but we also need to work on our physical being. If your health is not improving alongside your energy/spiritual journey, there is something that is being overlooked.

HEALING AND SPIRITUAL TOOLS: ACTIVATING SACRED GEOMETRY

I always thought sacred geometry meant the architectural knowledge applied to build a temple or sacred site. Little did I realize that the Creator has applied sacred geometry to all things great and small—the entire universe uses this principle. What does it mean for you?

It means that we have a universal God code or blueprint, and when this is without any interference or interruption, it manifests its full potential as healthy beings in harmony with the universal laws.

When discordant notes disturb the sacred geometry (emotions, trauma, etc.), then we experience challenges in health and life in general. There are many ways to activate your sacred geometry, or rather, get it to resonate clearly.

Meditation can do that, healing arts using sound-tuning forks, Tibetan Bowl music, harmonic frequencies like Solfeggio or crystals, esoteric acupuncture (an art form of acupuncture that works with needles, using sacred geometry patterns on the body), Sacred Activations offered by Tamra Oviatt, The Reconnection, Star Healing, biodynamic cranio-sacral therapy, and many other healing arts.

A simple and elegant way to activate sacred geometry is by using specifically researched tools that do that—to enhance health and life.

Sometimes loved ones have gone through surgery, can't swallow food or supplements, are in pain, or don't believe in getting help from a person. These are times when tools can be very handy and effective in healing and regeneration. There are a few well-researched and scientifically proven creations that do more than physical healing:

CONNECTING TO MOTHER EARTH

I was not sure in which chapter to mention Earthing or grounding. To me personally, this is a spiritual experience that trickles down to healing and health. I came across the book *Earthing: the most important health discovery.* Curiosity aroused, after an instant purchase, I devoured the book, and was amazed at all the science and research done on connecting to the Earth.

What does it mean? It means simply going barefoot in the grass, soil/ sand, or any conductive element like salt water.

The results of this are what astounded me:

» Dramatic reduction of any type of inflammation (seen as fast as in a few minutes)

» Better sleep to the point where people could give up medication

» Induces nervous system relaxation: reduces stress response by reducing cortisol and normalizing cortisol response

» Calming and reducing jet lag

» Reduction of allergies: environmental or food-type allergic reactions

» Dramatic pain reduction

» Harmonized women's hormones, reduced PMS, and menopausal symptoms

» Used by athletes for quick recovery

» Quickened healing times, often dramatic

» Sense of well being and security

» Boosts the immune system

» Better tempered children and adults

Connecting to our fundamental mother of all, the earth, is a profound feeling of "going back to the womb" for me. It creates a sense of well being, emotional and physical grounding, and tapping in to the abundance of healing that the earth freely provides.

If there is one thing to take away from this book—make earthing your prime choice, as it is so simple—as good as doing nothing.

You can purchase grounding sheets, mats, or inexpensive wrist bands to start getting grounded and connected, and feel the difference for yourself. You get the maximum output with the least effort. Love health short cuts!

One such tool is the **I.connect** and the **Heart Companion** pendant. These are either kept on the body, in a pocket, or worn on the person. They have shown to complete the auric field and improve the bio field of the person, create harmony around the person, and harmonize or activate sacred geometry in the person and their surroundings. It keeps the person "in the flow," so things manifest with ease rather than a struggle. It has even been proven to repair and regenerate organs and tissues. Gregory and Gail Hoag have researched this for over 30 years.

Another tool that has been confirmed to work on multiple levels for healing is Slim Spurling's **Light Life Technology Tools**—light life rings, harmonizers, feedback loops, and Acu Vac coils. If used correctly, they cannot only help pain and healing, but also help increase our own bio resonance fields, and increase our own consciousness.

DOS: The name is actually in Portugese, translated it means Systems Optimizer Disk.

This has been greatly researched (for 27 years), and through inspiration, developed by European Dr. Giampiero Cungi, in Brazil. These are a set of disks that need to be placed on different parts of the body. In layman's terms, it can instill permanent healing, harmonize dissonance in the body, and induce regeneration and positive growth. It uses quantum physics, mind-body medical science, and more, to create coherent information patterns, which when received by the body, start to stimulate a state of harmony and equilibrium at all levels.

RESOURCES
TO PURCHASE PRODUCTS

1. NUSKIN member signup: SG3011506 https://www.nuskin.com/content/nuskin/en_SG/home.html

2. CELERGEN (AVITA) member signup: SG844034[EO1] http://www.myavita.com/home.php

3. YOUNGEVITY member signup: 101397062 https://extranet.securefreedom.com/Youngevity/csSignup/EnrollNew_Ask.asp?ReturnURL=&Products=

4. IHERB.COM discount code: MAJ135 (. FOR GENERAL SUPPLEMENENTS, OHHIRA PROBIOTIC, ORGANIC PERSONAL CARE:)

5. JUENESSE GLOBAL website: www.bodybeautiful274.jeunesseglobal.com (FOR STEM CELL SKIN CARE)

6. FIT SOLUTION, member signup: BP 730568 https://fitsolutionsg.com/

7. YOUNGLIVING ESSENTIAL OILS enrolment number: 1116428 https://www.youngliving.com/en_SG

8. Dr Xeniji : https://www.elken.com/product_details.php?product_id=23

9.   Vielight : http://www.antiaging-nutrition.com/

10.   Microbiomax probiotic: info@infinitibiomed.com

11.   Thrive Level: https://le-vel.com/Products/THRIVE

12.   Deseret Biologicals: http://desbio.com/

13.   Earthing products: www.earthing.com

WEBSITES

1.   The Reconnection: http://www.thereconnection.com/

2.   Star Healing: http://kellyhamptononline.com/

3.   DOS: http://spiritofmaat.com/store/dos-discs/the-d-o-s-system/

4.   Mas Sajady: http://www.mas-sajady.com/

5.   Mashhur Anam: http://www.lifeharmonized.com/

6.   I Connect : http://iconnect2all.com/products/heartcompanion/

7.   Natural News : www.naturalnews.com

8.   Sacred Activations: http://sacredactivations.com/

9.   Julie Renee: http://julierenee.com/

10.   Veritalife: http://veritalife.com/

11.   Budwig: http://www.budwigcenter.com/the-budwig-diet/#.Ve-T4n_aqqko

12.   Light Life Technology Tools: http://www.lightlifetechnology.com/

13.   Jarrad Hewett: http://www.jarradhewett.com/

ABOUT THE AUTHOR

Sheeba Majmudar is a practicing nutritionist and naturopath who has been interviewed as an expert in her field by BBC Morning News.

She has mentored with some of the most experienced integrated doctors, like Dr. Kimberly Balas and Dr. Bruce Shelton, who are renowned as pioneers in their own fields, having forged new ways of thinking and doing.

Majmudar has applied these new ways of investigating to identify the root causes of a client's health issue(s) and recommending the relevant nutrients and therapies that have helped transform thousands of client's health's in a measurable, undisputable way—by improving clients' blood test results. This has allowed medical doctors to work with her with confidence. She has effectively bridged the medical world with the nutritional world, empowering clients to take one step at a time: taking them from multiple medications to none; from years of fertility challenges to natural pregnancies; from the pain of arthritis and fibromyalgia to a pain-free life; from the multitude of risks of obesity and toxicity to a transformed body and mind—wanting to eat right as a lifelong choice versus doing it occasionally.

The greatest learning or take-away from Majmudar is her ability to create awareness within the client that sparks their transformation, along with their own experience of improved health.

She herself is a passionate seeker of truth, and is always the curious student; her work is also her spiritual practice. She uses her intuition and her knack of being able to connect the dots, to work with the clients' psychology and help them to question their limited beliefs and push them to new levels of health and revelation—creating many "a-ha!" moments that click with them.

Always open to different techniques and ideas, she "cured" herself from childhood psoriasis, spondylitis, underactive thyroid, heavy metal toxicity, candida and leaky gut, food allergies and constant rhinitis, ovarian cysts, and frequent headaches, to now being completely free of all these challenges (despite getting older!), by using all the techniques mentioned in the book.

Majmudar walks her talk and lives the experience of this book in all aspects. Her work has reflected in her family's health, which has improved dramatically. The reason for her taking this journey is to seek better health the natural way. She is ever the student, seeking and learning new ways that enhance health, and is also a certified Herbalist, Aromatherapist, Reconnective Healer, and Cranio-sacral Therapist. She is also learned in Nutripuncture, Quantum Touch, Iridology, and Theta Healing. She continues her journey of discovery. She has a busy practice in Singapore, but works with clients all around the globe. Her website is www. sheebathenutritionist.com.

Printed in Great Britain
by Amazon